NUTRITION
FOR THE
DANCER

NUTRITION FOR THE DANCER

ZERLINA MASTIN

DANCE BOOKS • ALTON

First published in 2009 by Dance Books Ltd
The Old Bakery
4 Lenten Street
Alton
Hampshire GU34 1HG

ISBN 978 1 85273 135 9

A CIP catalogue record for this book is available
from the British Library

Produced by Jeremy Mills Publishing Ltd
www.jeremymillspublishing.co.uk

About the author

Zerlina Mastin gained a BA (Hons) at the Royal Academy of Dance, London, in 1999, and performed with various ballet and contemporary dance companies within the UK. She went on to study Nutrition and Dietetics at King's College London, graduating with a BSc in 2005. After working within the National Health Service, Zerlina turned to freelance nutrition consultation and journalism, specialising in sports nutrition and becoming a medical practitioner with Dance UK and the British Association of Performing Arts Medicine (BAPAM). *Nutrition for the Dancer* is her first book.

Acknowledgements

Thanks to Emma Heald, Emma Gibson, and Tirzah Mastin for providing the line illustrations.

Thanks also to the photographers and dancers whose work has enhanced this book. Their web site urls are:

Eric Richmond *www.erichmond.talktalk.net*
Phil Conrad *www.philconrad.net*
Rebecca Sewell (dancer) *www.longrunartistes.co.uk*
Kim Weston *www.kimweston.com*
Cassie Moore *www.am-london.com*
Kyle Stevenson *www.kylestevenson.com*

Contents

Prologue

The really great dancer is perhaps a rarer phenomenon than great musicians, painters or sculptors. This is because dance is a consummation of all these arts. The dancer, in addition to the qualities that pure dance demands, must be sensitive to and have an uncanny ear for music, must have a painter's sensibility to the significant line, a sculptor's approach to form, an architect's vision of space and a trained actor's responses to dramatic situations.

K. Subhas Chandran

To be able to dance is a wonderful gift, and a rare talent. It is where the essence, passion, spirit and beauty of the body are sculptured and choreographed through the movements of a dancer. The body is the instrument, and the dancer the artist.

To perform art, a dancer not only must be passionate, ambitious and doggedly determined to succeed, but must train and rehearse tirelessly to perfect technique, skill and stamina. And for the body to articulate the dancer's voice through the movement of its muscles, tendons, joints and ligaments, it needs an additional factor:

Food.

Food offers precious nutrients that enhance talent, unfold uniqueness and embellish character; and the immense value of food and the infinite quantity of nutrients it provides should never be underestimated or overlooked. When one wholeheartedly seeks to reach the extraordinary physical heights of a dancer, and can think of nothing more but pursuing a career and a life on stage, then talent and virtuosity is attained when, and only when, the body is respected.

Creatures who are dancers fit into societies all around the globe, and can be found in classical ballet companies warming up backstage in famous theatres, or glamorising theatres, films and television. There are dancers portraying the cultures of Asia, Africa and the Caribbean, professional ballroom dancers gracing our screens and ballrooms, and dancers capturing the intense curiosity of the media. There are choreographers creating movement, teachers inspiring pupils, movement therapists, notators, writers, historians, researchers and scientists. Dance and the celebration of dance permeate societies in every corner of the world.

The famous choreographer George Balanchine once said, 'One is born to be a dancer. No teacher can work miracles, nor will years of training make a good dancer of an untalented pupil.' Without talent, a dancer cannot succeed as a celebrated and recognised artist. Yet at the same time, talent and success do not come without tremendous pressure to maintain an ideal body shape: strong and lean muscles, immense flexibility, proportionate physique, svelte outline and considerably low body fat. So, many dancers are concerned about the delicate line between healthy living and a too-slender figure. Can a dancer remain extremely slim yet maintain a healthy diet and healthy body? Although each and every dancer is a unique individual, the answer to such a question is yes, most definitely.

There are innumerable reasons why a truly talented dancer is prevented from pursuing aspirations of a life on stage: discouragement from others about following a life in dance, the hurtful knock-backs experienced during auditioning, suffering from an injury, financial difficulties and personal circumstances are all factors that can put a halt or an abrupt end to a dancer's career.

Yet above all these reasons, nutrition could quite possibly be the biggest factor hindering a far greater number of dancers – a factor that has an immeasurable impact on dance students, professional dancers and dance culture as it continues to shape the artistic world. A diet targeting low body weight or a low fat percentage, or simply an unhealthy diet depleted of essential nutrients, is a hugely underestimated factor in the prevalence of injury, osteoporosis, amenorrhoea and low morale amongst dancers. The physical artistry of dance necessitates extraordinary physical athleticism, flexibility and strength that rival the same qualities in an athlete. Yet dance is also a performing art that seeks to portray beauty through the contours and physical form of the dancing body. The shape a dancer makes in space is synonymous with success as an artist.

To recognise the hurdles facing dancers during their career, a national enquiry administered and part-funded by Dance UK's 'Healthier Dancer Programme' consulted over a thousand dancers in the UK. The subsequent report discovered that 80 per cent of professional dancers experienced an average of three injuries each year. Of these dancers, 14 per cent were prevented from taking part in classes, rehearsals and performances for up to 18 months. Amenorrhoea (loss of menstruation) was experienced by 21 per cent of dancers for 6 months or more.

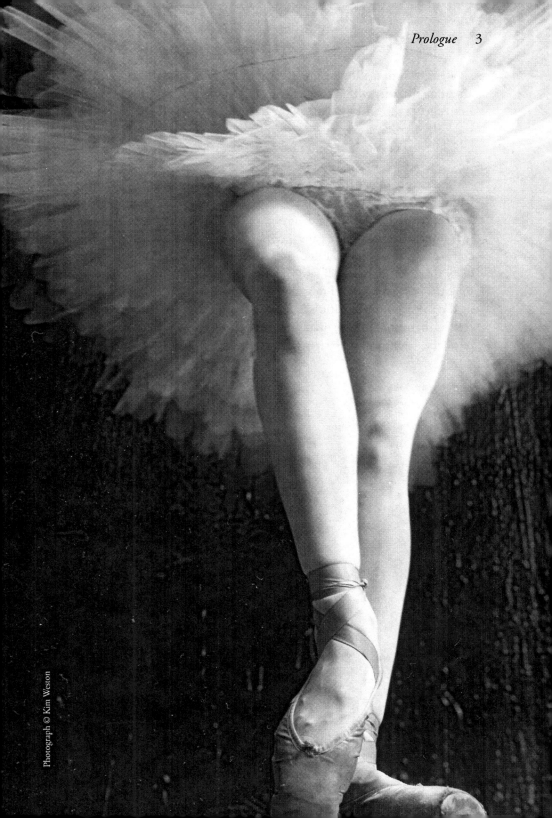

Results from the study also revealed that 16 per cent of dancers experienced an eating disorder within the previous 12 months, and 25 per cent had suffered from such a disorder at some point in their career. Taking into consideration the lack of professional nutritional advice tailored to a dancer's needs, one can only imagine the significant number of dancers who follow diets that compromise their strength, skill and, unquestionably, their talent.

The nature of dancing as a profession places a great deal of authority in the hands of teachers, choreographers, critics and audiences, meaning that dancers are highly vulnerable during their training and careers as artists. For that reason, it is imperative that they gain a sense of independence, self-sufficiency and control over their bodies. Educating dancers about nutrition and its impact on body shape and fitness will lead them to recognise the immense importance of their choice of foods, and most importantly, to feel empowered and confident in their decisions. Nutrition is a means to greater creativity and expression, rather than an obstacle that prevents dancers from achieving their ideal physique. This cannot be stressed enough.

Part 1
A Dancer's Diet

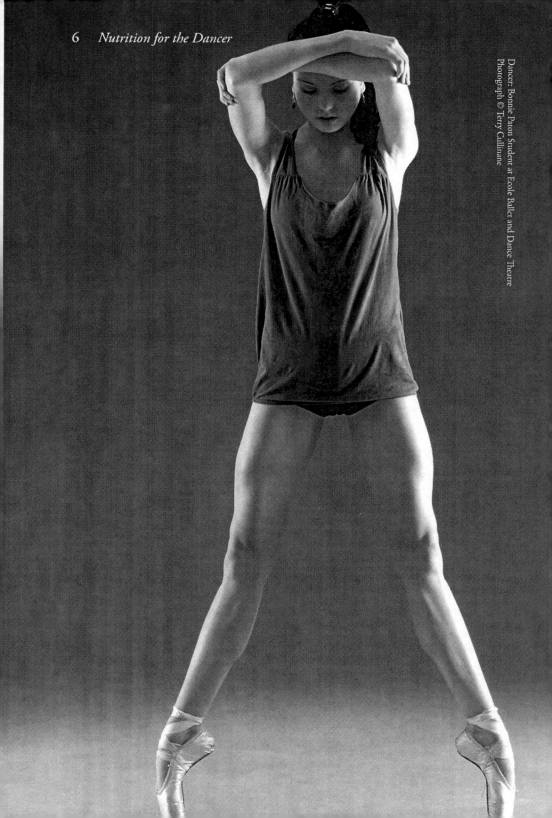

Chapter 1
Energy and the Calorie

> *Ballet dancing is arduous, strenuous activity. Students are engaged in*
> *physical training that rivals the training Olympic athletes undergo.*
> *At the same time, they strive for physical perfection not for the prowess*
> *alone but as a way of achieving the means necessary to express the*
> *pure nature of their art.*
>
> **George Balanchine**

Together, dance and science celebrate the extraordinary masterpiece that is the human body, and the way in which dancers express their art is made possible through the profound abilities of the human mind and the body. Science is the force behind the dancers' presence on stage, offering strength, flexibility and virtuosity to their movements. What comes after this is artistry: an affirmation of emotion, spontaneity, passion and psyche. So to understand where science meets the dancer, we journey back to the roots, or perhaps the seed, to where it all began: energy and the calorie – the science of food, and the life behind a dancer's shape in space.

The calorie – science meets the dancer

A calorie is simply a measure of energy. In scientific terms, 'energy' means 'ability to do work', whether it is energy from the breakdown of food, or energy produced from electricity, heat, light or other sources. 'Work' can be done using any of those forms of energy.

Energy in food is measured in kilojoules. When illustrated on food packages as 'Nutritional Information', the term *kilojoules* is abbreviated to *kJ*. Most people are more familiar with *kilocalories* (kcal), usually just referred to as *calories*.

To convert kJ to calories (kcal), simply divide by 4.2 (for example, 42kJ = 10kcal). To convert kcal to kJ, simply multiply by 4.2 (for example, 1kcal = 4.2kJ).

Example
An item of food has 1470kJ.
To convert to kcal: 1470kJ / 4.2 = 350 kcal

Retrieving energy from food: the digestive process

Once food enters the stomach, the process of digestion commences. Digestive enzymes (Figure 1) are minute substances made by the body to break down the food we eat. As food travels though the stomach, small intestine and large intestine, the body releases enzymes to break down nutrients within the meal. Once this process is complete, the many different nutrients are transported through the intestine wall and into the blood.

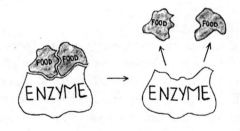

Figure 1. An enzyme

Calories: the body's fuel

We need energy to carry out a vast number of everyday activities, many of which we are unaware our bodies are performing. Energy from food is used to:

- maintain a steady body temperature
- fight infections and maintain a healthy immune system
- rebuild and repair cells (hair/skin/organs)
- feed the most important organ – the brain
- allow the lungs to take up oxygen during breathing
- support the heart when it contracts and forces blood around the body
- make movements (such as walking, shopping, showering)
- dance.

Thus energy in the form of calories is necessary even when we are not moving at all. Dancing can increase our daily energy requirements by 25–75 per cent, depending on exercise frequency, intensity and metabolic rate.

Calculating your nutritional requirements

Before determining your own personal calorie requirements, you should study the following terms so that you can understand the numbers obtained from the final calculations.

- **Metabolic rate** – the rate or speed at which our bodies use energy (calories). Metabolic rate is affected by exercise, eating habits, how much muscle we have, genetic makeup and our general health.
- **RMR (resting metabolic rate)** – how many calories are needed when you are motionless (lying down but not sleeping).
- **DEE (daily energy expenditure)** – how many calories are needed for everyday movement (walking to and from work, shopping etc.), excluding any form of exercise.
- **TEE (total energy expenditure)** – the total number of calories required for daily activities AND exercise (such as rehearsals, dance classes and performances).

To calculate your requirements, you will first need to know your weight in kilograms (kg). The following example demonstrates how to convert from stones (st) and pounds (lb) to kilograms.

> **Example**
> A dancer weighing 8 stone and 9 pounds (abbreviated to 8st and 9lb).
> **Step 1.** Convert st into lb (there are 14 lb in a stone).
> 8st × 14 = 112lb
> **Step 2.** Add the remaining 9 lb.
> 112lb + 9lb = 121lb
> **Step 3.** Convert lb into kg (by dividing by 2.2).
> 121lb / 2.2 = 55kg

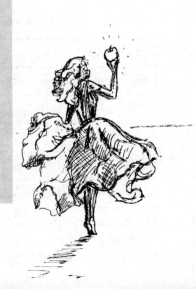

Calculating your resting metabolic rate (RMR)

RMR = Bodyweight (kg) × 14.7 + 496

Example
A dancer weighing 55kg.
55kg × 14.7 + 496 = 1305kcal
Resting metabolic rate (RMR) = **1305kcal**

Calculating your daily energy expenditure (DEE)

This estimates the number of calories needed to do basic day-to-day activities.
DEE = RMR × 1.4

Example
The same dancer.
1305kcal × 1.4 = 1827kcal
Daily energy expenditure (DEE) = **1827kcal**

NOTE: If you are injured and mainly sitting, use DEE = RMR × 1.2

Calculating your total energy expenditure (TEE)

First add up how many classes, rehearsals and performances you take in a week. Table 1.1 estimates the number of calories burnt in several different styles of dance. Note that these values will vary depending on weight, age, metabolic rate and fitness levels.

Table 1.1. Different dance styles and energy expenditure

Style of dance	Kcal burnt per hour (approx.)
Ballet – moderate intensity	300
Ballet – high intensity	480
Pilates	210
Contemporary – medium intensity	300
Contemporary – high intensity	480
Musical theatre (combination of low/high intensity)	480

Tango – moderate intensity	350
Pointe work – technique classes	250
Irish dancing	450
Performance	Add up total hours spent performing, and calculate depending on exercise intensity

Example
Our dancer is involved in 7 classes, 2 rehearsals and 2 performances each week.

Total 1hr classes in a week: 7 (7 × 300kcal = 2100kcal)
Total 1hr rehearsals in a week: 2 (2 × 300 kcal = 800kcal)
Total performances in a week: 2 (2 × 600kcal = 1200kcal)
Total calories used in these: 2100 + 800 + 1200 = 4100kcal per week

In order to put all these calculations together, we first need to calculate calorie requirements for a week, then divide this by 7 to work out how many calories are needed for 1 day. Other than taking a few extra snacks when training hard, it is better to eat roughly the same amount each day, as the body works better with regular eating patterns, and it encourages a healthy metabolic rate.

Example
Our dancer's daily energy expenditure (DEE) is 1827 kcal.
Calorie requirements for a week: 1827kcal × 7 = 12,789kcal
Calories required for dance rehearsals and classes for a week = 4100kcal
Adding these two figures gives us the dancer's total energy expenditure (TEE) for a week (how much energy is required for everyday activities and exercise).
Total energy expenditure for a week: 12,789kcal + 4100kcal = 16,889kcal
TEE for 1 day = 16,889kcal / 7 = **2412 kcal per day**
Therefore our dancer, who weighs 55kg and has 7 classes, 2 rehearsals and 2 performances each week, needs around 2400kcal every day to maintain a steady weight and have enough energy to perform at an optimal level.

It is interesting to calculate how much of your personal daily calorie requirements is needed for dance.

Example
Using the results calculated above for our dancer, the percentage required for normal life is

$$\frac{12789\text{kcal} - 4100\text{kcal}}{12789} \times 100$$

Percentage of calories required for *non*-dancing activities = 67%
Therefore, percentage of calories needed to dance = 100% − 67% = 33%.
So dancing took up 33% (a third) of the dancer's total calorie requirements.

Summary

- Calories represent the energy we find in the food we eat, and the measures that we use for it are kJ (kilojoules) and kcal (kilocalories).
- Enzymes break down the food we eat, and the nutrients within the food are then transported to every cell in our bodies to be used for energy or other purposes.
- Almost every activity within the body needs energy. We need energy to keep our bodies at a perfect 36.5°C, energy to help our lungs take up oxygen, energy for the brain, and energy to provide working muscles when dancing.
- Metabolic rate is the speed at which our bodies use up energy to survive. This energy comes from the food we eat and from our own body's reserves. Our individual metabolic rates can be affected by how fit we are, our eating habits and our genetic makeup.
- Resting metabolic rate (RMR) is the minimum number of calories needed to maintain ourselves (lying down but not sleeping).
- Daily energy expenditure (DEE) is the total number of calories that we need when going about everyday activities such as walking, shopping and showering.
- Total energy expenditure (TEE) is the total number of calories we need to live, walk around and also take part in dance classes, rehearsals and performances.

Chapter 2
The Macronutrients

Part 1
Carbohydrate

When I miss class for one day, I know it.
When I miss class for two days, my teacher knows it.
When I miss class for three days, the audience knows it.

Rudolf Nureyev

Chapter 1 showed how to calculate your daily energy requirements. If this gives you a total that is notably at variance with your present diet, now is the perfect time to make a change! These calculations act as a guideline for estimating how many calories you need during intense exercise, during rest, or when managing an injury. On the odd occasion, you may want to calculate your daily calorie intake by keeping a 24-hour food diary. This will give you a general idea as to whether you are eating the right amount for what you are trying to achieve.

The next three chapters look at the main food groups that constitute the dancer's diet: carbohydrate, protein and fat.

When added together, carbohydrate, protein and fat represent your daily calorie needs as estimated in Chapter 1. It is particularly important to balance these macronutrients in the right proportion to each other, as they have very specific roles within the body (Figure 2).

Figure 2. Carbohydrate, protein and fat: the balance of macronutrients in the dancer's diet

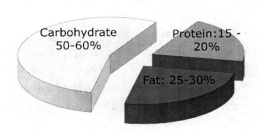

The concentrations of energy in these three macronutrients are not all the same:

1 gram of carbohydrate (CHO) = 4kcal
1 gram of protein = 4kcal
1 gram of fat = 9kcal

As protein, fat and carbohydrate have different energy concentrations, the foods we eat have different calorie contents because foods are made up of different amounts of carbohydrate, protein and fat. Here's an example. Both these snacks weigh 40 grams, but have quite different calorie contents.

Example

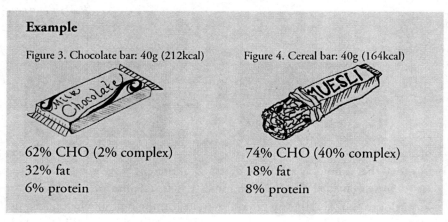

Figure 3. Chocolate bar: 40g (212kcal)   Figure 4. Cereal bar: 40g (164kcal)

62% CHO (2% complex)   74% CHO (40% complex)
32% fat   18% fat
6% protein   8% protein

The importance of carbohydrate for the dancer

If you're spending all your waking hours practising in the dance studio, and have counted triple figures on the number of times you have rehearsed that tedious leg move, you may be forgiven for missing out on the fervour surrounding the subject of carbohydrate: too much? not enough? wrong timing? on an empty stomach?

For a dancer, carbohydrate is not only a source of energy. It also has a very important role as a nutrient, because it:

- helps to burn fat when exercising
- prevents the body from using protein from muscle
- provides a host of B vitamins that boost metabolism
- prevents fatigue and heavy, tired muscles
- prevents injury caused by exhausted muscles and vulnerable joints, ligaments and bones.

Simple and complex carbohydrates

There are two types of carbohydrate: complex (starch and fibre) and simple (sugar). The words 'complex' and 'simple' reflect the size of the carbohydrate molecule.

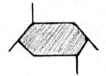

Figure 5. Sugar molecule   Figure 6. Starch molecule

Complex carbohydrates (starch and fibre) are broken down into simple sugars by digestive enzymes. These nutrients then pass through the intestine wall and into the blood to be used by the body.

Table 2.1 shows examples of carbohydrate sources in food.

Some foods have a single type, others a combination of simple and complex carbohydrates.

Table 2.1. Examples of carbohydrate sources in food

Foods high in complex carbohydrates (starch and fibre)	Foods high in simple carbohydrates (sugar)	A combination of simple and complex carbohydrates (sugar, starch and fibre)
Pasta	Sugar (brown and white)	Whole fruit (fresh, tinned
Rice	Honey, jam, marmalade and	in natural juice, dried,
Potatoes, sweet potatoes,	other preserves	frozen)
yams	Fruit (flesh eaten without	Sweet pastries, pies and flans
Bread (loaf, pitta, bagel,	the skin)	Biscuits
bread rolls, chapatti,	Soft drinks	Cakes
white/brown/wholemeal)	Milk	
Noodles	Ice cream	
Couscous	Yoghurt	
Flour (brown and white)	Jelly	
Oats	Fromage frais	
Other grains	Sweets and confectionery	
Breakfast cereals	Glucose tablets	
(unsweetened)		
Pulses (beans, lentils, peas)		
Plantains (green bananas)		
Parsnips		
Sweetcorn		

Glycogen – what is it?

The body holds a small amount of carbohydrate in muscle, and this is stored as glycogen. Glycogen is very similar in structure to complex carbohydrate, and is made up of many sugar molecules joined together. The amount of glycogen our muscles can store is equivalent to 1600–2000kcal, only enough to last 24 hours if we were to eat nothing.

The effect of glycogen levels on performance

During exercise, muscle glycogen levels gradually fall, and on average we have enough glycogen to fuel 90–180 minutes of moderate activity. As these levels become progressively lower, the body sends signals to the brain telling it to either stop exercising or slow down. How does the body let us know if we fail to slow down or stop? We become tired, our movements become sluggish and difficult to perform, and our technique suffers. Poise, balance and artistry are also affected, and all because we have simply run out of glycogen.

Why does carbohydrate help to burn fat?

You cannot drive a car without fuel. Similarly, fat cannot be burned without the presence of carbohydrate either in our food or stored in our muscles (as glycogen). Muscles will first use carbohydrate to fuel a dance class or rehearsal; then, depending on fitness levels, they will switch to using both carbohydrate and fat.

As fitness levels increase, enzymes responsible for breaking down fat for energy become more efficient, meaning that more fat is burnt and we enjoy greater energy and stamina levels, as vital glycogen stores in muscle are not rapidly depleted. Fatigue is kept at bay. In trained dancers undertaking moderate to high-intensity exercise, fat can be used as a source of fuel after 15 minutes.

Why does carbohydrate prevent the body from using protein in muscle?

If we eat sufficient amounts of carbohydrate before dancing, glycogen levels are topped up, and our muscles then use glycogen and fat for energy. If we have not eaten enough carbohydrate, the body runs low on glycogen, and it finds it much harder to burn fat. Muscles will be forced to use another source of energy – protein. And unlike the situation with fat and carbohydrate, we do not have extra stores of protein. Although small amounts of protein are used for energy during exercise, *three times* more protein is used when glycogen levels are low. Losing muscle not only results in loss of strength and stamina, but also reduces the metabolic rate. Far more calories are needed to maintain muscle than to maintain fat; therefore if we have less muscle, we need fewer calories.

How much carbohydrate should we eat, and which type is the healthiest?

Carbohydrate contributes around 50–60 per cent of the dancer's daily diet. So, to ensure you include enough, base each meal and snack around a source of carbohydrate (aim to fill a third of your plate with a carbohydrate-rich food such as rice, pasta, potatoes, couscous or equivalent).

One type of carbohydrate is not necessarily considered better or healthier than another. All carbohydrates are broken down into simple carbohydrates during digestion, and so the most suitable type of carbohydrate really depends on how quickly we need that energy. Some carbohydrates are absorbed much more quickly than others, and are used more rapidly by working muscles.

However, things are not quite as straightforward as thinking that simple sugars reach muscles more quickly, and that complex sugars take more time because they first need to be broken down. Many starchy foods such as bread and potatoes can be digested and absorbed quite rapidly. Also, fruits such as apples are high in simple carbohydrates, yet they release energy moderately slowly because they also contain fibre, which slows down digestion.

So what should you aim for? To simply maximise stamina, skill and performance, keeping blood sugars stable is the key. If blood sugars continually rise and fall, consequences include erratic energy levels, inconsistent performance, exhaustion and low mood. Additionally, rebellious blood sugars encourage sugar cravings – cue empty sweet packets and uncontrollable blood sugars.

What to eat before and after a dance class, rehearsal or performance

What and how much you choose to eat will have an enormous impact on your performance, skill, execution of steps and artistry. The appropriate amount to eat depends on the duration and intensity of the dance class or performance (for example, a smaller, less demanding class will require less carbohydrate). To calculate your exact carbohydrate requirements, refer to Appendix 8, 'Calculations'.

Preparation – eating before training

Before training, the stomach needs a certain amount of time to settle and feel comfortable. When we eat, blood rushes to the stomach to digest food and transport it to working muscles. This can involve up to 30 per cent of our total blood volume. Thus to avoid discomfort and ensure that muscles have a good supply of blood, aim to leave at least 30 minutes between eating and training.

Every dancer varies the timing of meals and snacks, but generally you should try to eat meals 2 to 4 hours before training. After a small snack, leave around 30 minutes to 2 hours before training. Clearly the precise timing of your meal or snack may depend on schedules and food available, but you will know through experience the best time to eat and train.

Meals and snacks for the dancer

To be fully prepared for a dance class or performance, you need to make sure that your muscle glycogen levels are topped up. That means basing a meal on a carbohydrate. The following meal and snack ideas are good sources of carbohydrate and are all naturally low in fat. Some of the meals are very quick and easy to prepare.

2 to 4 hours before dancing

- Wholegrain cereal (e.g. Weetabix, bran or wheat flakes, muesli) made with skimmed milk or low-fat yoghurt
- Porridge made with skimmed milk and a small handful of raisins
- Sandwich/bagel/pitta/roll/wrap filled with sliced chicken, fish, egg or quorn (using low-fat cream cheese instead of butter)
- Jacket potato with beans/tuna & tomato sauce/chicken/cream or cottage cheese. No butter
- Pasta in tomato sauce with grated low-fat cheese and vegetables
- Prawn/chicken/tofu/quorn stir-fry with vegetables and noodles or rice (accompanied by a low-fat dressing or sauce)
- Fish and potato pie (see recipe, page 137)
- Bean hotpot with rice (see recipe, page 140)
- Couscous with lemon chicken and vegetables.

Snacks: 30 minutes to 2 hours before dancing

- Fresh fruit
- Dried fruit (apricots, dates and raisins)
- Diluted fruit juice
- Smoothie
- Shake (home-made or meal replacement)
- Cereal/energy bar
- Low-fat yoghurt
- Fruit loaf/raisin bread
- Handful of mixed fruit and nuts.

Sugary foods and drinks before training

Sugary foods and drinks eaten before any sort of exercise can be a little risky if the timing is inaccurate, or if you are particularly sensitive to changes in your blood sugar levels.

Sugary foods and drinks produce a rapid rise in blood sugar, but also a rapid dip afterwards. During this short-lived dip, you could experience the effects of low blood sugars (poor energy levels, light-headedness, nausea, heavy muscles, difficulty in concentrating), and exercises would feel difficult to perform well.

To prevent this from occurring, the safest option is to consume a meal or snack that releases energy more slowly, as listed above.

During training

If training lasts less than an hour, water is fine to drink if you have eaten sufficient quantities of carbohydrate during the previous few days and eaten a meal rich in carbohydrate 2–4 hours before training.

When you train for more than an hour at a moderate to high intensity, carbohydrate will help delay fatigue caused by depleted glycogen levels. If the exercise involves fast, rapid or dynamic movements, sharp and frequent changes of direction, and lifts, then it is likely that your training is of high intensity. Remember that it is important to consume a source of carbohydrate before fatigue sets in.

If you train for a considerable amount of time at a moderate to high intensity and without taking a break, your body will not be able to keep blood sugars and glycogen at optimal levels. This is because your muscles can use only a certain amount of carbohydrate in a given time, and therefore consuming more than this will not improve your energy levels or help you burn fat.

Table 2.2 provides details on suitable snacks and drinks during exercise. Depending on the length and intensity of exercise, choose between the two values given. Whether you choose a drink or a food is a matter of preference, as both work equally well. If you choose to eat something, then make sure that you drink some water too.

Table 2.2. Food and drink to consume during class/rehearsal or performance

Food or drink	Minimum	Moderate to high-intensity training
Energy bar (sports)	1 bar	1–2 bars
Bananas	1–2 bananas	2–3 bananas
Raisins or sultanas	1 handful (50g)	2 handfuls (100g)
Cereal bar	1 bar	2 bars
Diluted fruit juice (50% water, 50% juice)	500ml	1000ml
Cereal (eg sultana bran)	1 handful (40g)	2 handfuls (80g)
Oatcakes	3	6
Isotonic sports drink (6g per 100ml)	500ml	1000ml

After exercise

Once the class or performance is over, refuelling should take priority. The length and intensity of the class, and the quantity of carbohydrate consumed before exercise, will have a direct impact on how quickly you can restock.

Did you know?
It can take up to 20 hours to replace glycogen stores after moderate to high-intensity exercise.

The most effective time to start refuelling is as soon as possible after training – ideally, within 2 hours after exercise. The following post-exercise snacks also provide a good source of protein (protein is discussed in Chapter 3).

- 1–2 cartons of yoghurt
- 1–2 portions of fresh fruit with a glass of skimmed or semi-skimmed milk
- Yoghurt drink
- Sports bar (must contain both carbohydrate and protein)
- Sandwich/bagel/wrap/pitta with lean meat/poultry/egg/tuna
- Meal-replacement shake
- Jacket potato with tuna/baked beans or grated low fat cheddar cheese
- Healthy bowl of cereal and skimmed/semi-skimmed milk.

Try to avoid eating large and infrequent meals or lots of sugary snacks, as this may produce large fluctuations in blood sugar levels and will also result in periods of time when muscle glycogen will be low. Frequent rises in blood sugars may also encourage the body to store more energy as fat (see Chapter 4). You should aim to have smaller and more frequent meals and snacks that ensure a steady supply of carbohydrate.

Why does the body hold water when I eat a carbohydrate-rich meal?

Three grams of water is needed to store one gram of glycogen in muscle, and therefore a small weight gain can be noted on the scales when carbohydrate-rich foods are consumed. However, it is not all gloom and dismay; there are several very important reasons why this is beneficial.

Firstly, glycogen is needed to fuel dance exercises and training in order to maximise stamina and execution of steps, and also to keep fatigue and injury at bay. Additionally, the body needs glycogen to enable it to produce energy from fat, thus helping to keep the body trim and toned. As glycogen in muscle is slowly used up during exercise, water is lost with it, and body weight goes back to normal. So not only have you had a good training session and used fat for energy, but you have also kept your energy levels high.

How can I avoid feeling heavy after eating a carbohydrate meal?

Some dancers experience a general heaviness of the body following a meal containing carbohydrate. The following tips should help alleviate these symptoms at the same time as ensuring that your diet still contains adequate amounts of carbohydrate.

- Try to space out your meals and snacks evenly so that you are not eating a lot before exercise.
- Try not to eat anything too bulky (high in fibre) before exercise.
- Leave sufficient time between eating and exercising.
- Ensure you drink plenty of fluids.

Fibre – a complex carbohydrate

Fibre is a complex carbohydrate found in cereals, fruits and vegetables. It is not digested, but instead helps maintain a healthy digestive tract. For a dancer, fibre can:

- add bulk to meals, thus helping to control body weight
- keep bowels healthy and combat constipation
- slow down the absorption of sugar from the digestive tract into the blood, thus preventing fluctuating blood sugar levels (fluctuating blood sugars not only affect energy levels and performance, but can also encourage weight gain and fat storage)
- help control appetite.

Soluble and insoluble fibre

There are two types of fibre, soluble and insoluble, and foods can contain either or both. Insoluble fibre is completely indigestible, and is found in bran, fruits, vegetables and wholegrain products. It is slightly heavier than soluble fibre, but adds bulk to foods and helps to maintain healthy bowels.

Soluble fibre is used as a source of fuel by bacteria in the gut. It also adds bulk to foods, but is slightly kinder and lighter on the digestive system. Soluble fibre is found in oats, fruits and vegetables, beans and pulses.

Including more fibre in the diet

Here are some tips on increasing the amount of fibre in your diet. Introduce high-fibre foods gradually – your body needs time to adjust, and you may experience some abdominal discomfort if you overdo it at first.

- Choose wholegrain bread, wholemeal pitta, brown rice and pasta.
- Aim for 5–7 portions of fruit and vegetables each day.
- Choose a wholemeal breakfast cereal such as porridge or one based on wheat or bran.
- Add beans and pulses to meat dishes and salads.

Tip
When including more fibre in the diet, ensure that you include plenty of fluids.

Chapter summary

- Carbohydrate, protein and fat are the three main components that make up our diet. Carbohydrate contributes around 50–60 per cent of our daily intake.
- These three macronutrients vary in their energy content: carbohydrate and protein contain 4kcal for each gram, and fat 9kcal per gram.
- Carbohydrate's main role is to provide energy, which is used to fuel almost every activity occurring within the body.
- The two types of carbohydrates are known as simple carbohydrate (sugar) and complex carbohydrate (starch and fibre). Complex carbohydrate is made up of many sugar molecules joined together.
- Foods can have a single type of carbohydrate or both types.
- A small amount of carbohydrate is stored as glycogen in muscle. These stores provide energy for peak performance, help burn fat during exercise, and prevent early fatigue, heavy tired muscles and injury.
- When glycogen stores become low, less fat is burned and muscles use three times as much protein as when glycogen levels are high.
- Aim to eat carbohydrates regularly and with each meal to keep muscle glycogen levels topped up. Try to eat a meal 2 to 4 hours before exercise and/or a small snack 30 minutes to 2 hours before training.

- The ideal carbohydrate intake will vary according to your level of training – the longer and more intense it is, the more carbohydrate you require.
- If training lasts more than an hour, and its intensity is moderate to high, aim to consume a source of carbohydrate before fatigue sets in.
- The most effective time to replenish muscle glycogen levels is within 2 hours after training.

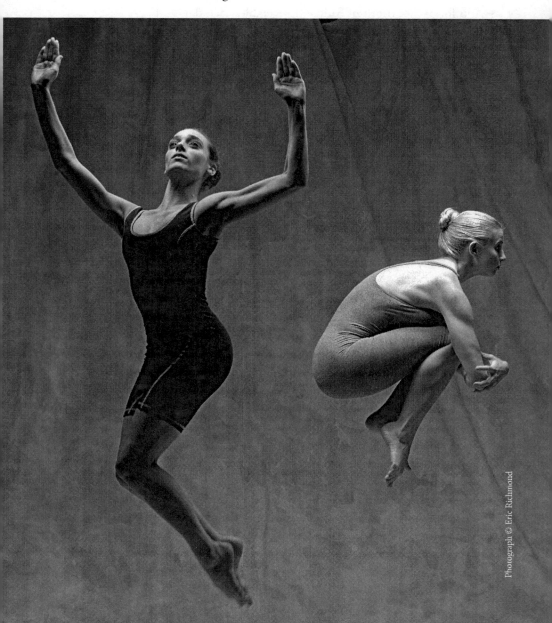

Photograph © Eric Richmond

Chapter 3
The Macronutrients

Part 2

Protein

Dancing appears glamorous, easy, delightful. But the path to paradise of the achievement is not easier than any other. There is fatigue so great that the body cries, even in its sleep. There are times of complete frustration, there are daily small deaths.

Martha Graham

Before reading this chapter, you may be forgiven for presuming that protein is necessary only for those pursuing trouser-splitting quadriceps, or dreaming of becoming the next Popeye impersonator. Admittedly, such thinking does hold a grain of truth (!), but protein is part of every single cell, and is vital in enabling the body to repair, grow and maintain itself.

Protein contributes around 15 to 20 per cent of our calorie requirements each day, and can be used as a source of energy because muscle cells have enzymes capable of breaking down all three macronutrients (although it is more difficult for the body to convert protein into energy). Using protein for energy, however, is certainly not something desirable for a dancer, because, in addition, dietary protein:

- plays a vital role in achieving balance, poise, core strength and grace by maintaining and building muscles attached to bone (skeletal muscle)
- prevents water retention
- prevents injury caused by lack of supporting muscle
- encourages healthy hair and skin.

Healthy cells and tissue are constantly renewed, as they are continually broken down and replaced by new tissue. A regular supply of protein is imperative, because a lack of protein in the diet would mean loss of muscle, strength and skill. But protein also has another important mission: to enhance the dancer's future as a performer.

Building bulky muscles is not something the average dancer desires, as it can restrict movement, flexibility and the ability to create elongated lines through long lean muscles. Male dancers may desire greater muscle mass for aesthetics, for strength to execute high leaps and turns, and also to lift the female dancer and support her movements. Although a dancer may not wish to have bulky muscles, protein is still extremely important in dance; it requires a tremendous amount of strength and stamina to execute virtuosic movements, or to hold applause-worthy balances on *pointe*!

Table 3.1 lists some protein-rich foods. These are further divided into categories (meat and fish, dairy products and eggs, grains and cereals, pulses, nuts and seeds, soya products, other), and the table gives guidelines on portion sizes.

Table 3.1. Protein-rich foods

Food	Portion size	Protein per portion (g)
Meat and fish		
Tuna in brine	1 small tin (100g)	24
Haddock (baked)	1 fillet (140g)	32
Salmon (grilled)	1 fillet (150g)	30
Beef fillet (grilled/lean)	2 slices (105g)	31
Chicken breast (grilled)	1 breast (130g)	38
Turkey (roasted)	2 slices (140g)	41
Dairy products and eggs		
Skimmed milk	150ml	5
Semi-skimmed milk	150ml	5
Low-fat yoghurt (plain)	1 carton (150g)	8
Low-fat yoghurt (fruit)	1 carton (150g)	6
Fromage frais	1 small carton (100g)	7
Cheese (cheddar – reduced fat)	1 thick slice (40g)	13
Cottage cheese	1 small carton (110g)	15
Eggs	1 large	8

Food	Portion size	Protein per portion (g)
Grains and cereals		
Wholemeal bread	2 slices	7.5
White bread	2 slices	6.5
Brown rice (boiled)	1 bowl (180g)	5
White rice (boiled)	1 bowl (180g)	5
Pasta (boiled)	1 bowl (180g)	5.5
Egg noodles (boiled)	1 bowl (180g)	4
Pulses		
Baked beans	1 small tin (200g)	10
Red kidney beans (boiled)	3 tbsp (120g)	9
Black Eye Beans	3 tbsp (120g)	8
Chickpeas (boiled)	3 tbsp (120g)	12
Nuts and seeds		
Peanuts – roasted + salted	1 handful (50g)	12
Peanut butter	20g	5
Pecan nuts	1 handful	5
Sunflower seeds	2 tbsp (30g)	6
Sesame seeds	2 tbsp (25g)	4
Soya products		
Soya milk	1 glass (150ml)	5
Soya mince	2 tbsp – before cooking	11
Tofu	½ pack (100g)	8
Other		
Quorn mince	4 tbsp (100g)	12

Protein and digestion: science meets the dancer again

We can compare the structure of protein to that of carbohydrate. Rather than being made up of lots of small sugar molecules, protein is made up of a long chain of *amino acids* (see Figure 7).

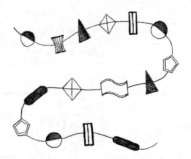

Figure 7. A chain of amino acids

There are twenty different amino acids in total, which can be combined in many ways to form hundreds of different proteins.

During digestion, protein is broken down into amino acids by digestive enzymes. Amino acids supplied through the diet are then reassembled back into various proteins, depending on what the body needs.

The body is capable of making twelve out of the twenty amino acids, and so these twelve are known as *non-essential* (meaning that it is not essential to have them in our diet). The remaining eight cannot be made by the body, and therefore must come from the foods we eat. These amino acids are called *essential* (refer to Appendix 7 for a list of the essential and non-essential amino acids).

Fish, poultry, red meat, eggs, dairy products and soya products contain all twenty amino acids, and so these foods are considered to be of *high biological value* or *complete* (very good quality protein!). Some foods not of animal origin do not contain all twenty amino acids; this applies to vegetable sources of protein listed in Table 3.1. Foods that do not provide all twenty are termed of *lower biological value* or *incomplete*. Dancers following a vegetarian diet need simply to follow a well-balanced diet that includes a variety of different plant-based foods (i.e., choose foods from each of the different food groups in Table 3.1). This will ensure that their diet includes adequate amounts of protein.

Estimating your protein requirements

It has been well documented that dancers require more dietary protein than the general population does: not only do dancers have a greater percentage of lean muscle that needs to be maintained, but dancing increases the speed with which muscle is broken down and rebuilt.

Your individual protein requirements depend on the type of training you undertake, how intense it is, and what you are aiming to achieve.

Table 3.2: Protein requirements for dancers

Type of exercise	Daily protein requirements per kg of body weight
For optimal performance	1.2–1.6g
Dancer on muscle-gain programme	1.8–2.0g
Dancer on weight-loss programme	1.6–2.0g

NOTE: All dance styles require similar amounts of protein.

> **Example**
> A ballet dancer weighing 55kg, with 4 dance classes per week.
> 55kg × 1.2g/kg = 66g per day
> 55kg × 1.6g/kg = 88g per day
> Daily protein requirement = **66–88g**

How to ensure you include enough protein in your diet

If you are meeting your calorie requirements and are including 2–4 servings of protein-rich foods each day (a meat or fish serving that takes up around a third of your plate), then it is likely that you are meeting your protein requirements too (see Table 3.1 for portion sizes). If you reduce your calorie intake, it will be more difficult to maintain an adequate protein intake (remember, you also need sufficient amounts of carbohydrate in your diet to ensure that your body doesn't use protein for energy).

If you are following a weight loss programme, you require a slightly higher protein intake to ensure that weight loss is restricted to fat rather than muscle. Animal sources of protein are good choices, so simply choose lean cuts of meat and low-fat dairy options.

Is too much protein harmful?

Eating more protein than you need will not offer any benefit in health or performance. Additional protein cannot be converted into muscle or increase stamina or strength; your body is able to use only a certain amount of protein each day to build and maintain muscle.

A small excess of dietary protein is unlikely to be converted into fat. Weight gain as fat is predominantly caused by excessive calories and a high-fat diet. A significant percentage of calories supplied by protein is given off as heat, and having adequate amounts of protein in the diet has actually been shown to improve the metabolic rate.

Previous thinking assumed that excess protein was damaging to the liver and kidneys. It was also thought that too much protein caused the body to excrete large amounts of calcium, an important mineral necessary for strong bones. In healthy people, however, this theory has not been demonstrated, and therefore eating too much protein is unlikely to be harmful.

Importance of consuming protein after exercise

During a class or performance, your muscles work extremely hard not only to support the movement of skeletal bones during challenging dance sequences, but also to protect your bones from injury and continually improve your technique, skill and poise. Therefore the best time to refuel tired muscles is within the first 2 hours after training. By combining protein and carbohydrate in a meal or snack after training, you will be promoting good muscle definition and tone, and keeping muscle glycogen levels at an optimal level. The post-exercise snacks listed in Chapter 2 provide an ideal combination of protein and carbohydrate whilst also being low in fat.

Chapter summary

- Protein is continually broken down and rebuilt in a dancer's body to maintain healthy cells and tissues.
- Dietary protein not only builds skeletal muscle, but also develops poise, balance, grace and skill.
- Twenty different amino acids make up the structure of protein. Eight are essential (are not made naturally by the body) and must be included in our diet.

- Foods of animal origin (red meat, poultry, fish, eggs, dairy products) have a complete protein profile, as they contain all twenty amino acids. Include two to four portions of low-fat sources of protein each day.
- Vegetarian diets can easily provide adequate amounts of protein if a variety of protein-rich plant-based foods and low-fat dairy products are included.
- For optimal performance, you should aim for 1.2–1.6g of protein per kg of bodyweight. If you are following a weight loss programme, 1.6–2.0g of protein per kg of bodyweight is required. To gain muscle mass, 1.8–2.0g is suggested.
- Consuming protein (in combination with carbohydrate) in the first 2 hours after training will help promote lean, toned muscles.
- Evidence does not suggest that too much protein is harmful in healthy individuals.
- A diet rich in protein has been shown to improve the metabolic rate.

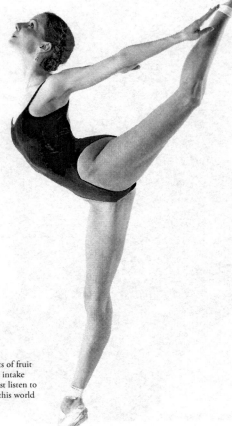

Dancer: Rebecca Sewell 'I try to stay healthy, eating lots of fruit and vegetables and consciously try to increase my fluid intake throughout the day. It's important for me to try and just listen to my body more, especially trying to live and survive in this world environment every day that we do!'
Photograph © Phil Conrad

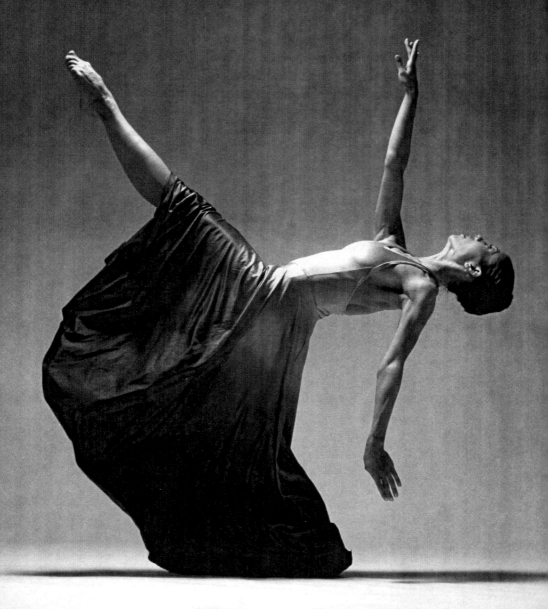

Chapter 4
The Macronutrients

Part 3

Fat

The devil has put a penalty on all things we enjoy in life.
Either we suffer in health ... we suffer in soul ... or we get fat.

Albert Einstein

Unfortunately, fat is hidden in so many everyday foods available in supermarkets, corner shops, canteens, restaurants and cafes that it is rather difficult to avoid or limit. Processed foods, fast foods, desserts and sweets are all high in fat (and unhealthy fat, moreover). And because fat is dense in energy (9 kcal per gram compared with 4 kcal per gram in carbohydrate and protein), it can quite easily lead to weight gain.

Despite its lack of popularity and long-standing faithful friends, fat is a vital part of a dancer's diet. Each single healthy cell requires fat as part of its structure, and fat is involved in every activity within the body. It should, however, only contribute around 25 per cent of your diet, so a low-fat diet is, unfortunately, a must!

This chapter gives advice on how to follow a low-fat diet whilst still ensuring that it includes the important fats that are vital for a dancer. And furthermore, this chapter will illustrate that low fat doesn't mean we have to swap chocolate bars for celery sticks or cabbage soup ...

Why do we need fat in our diets?

Here are just a few of the ways in which fat contributes to the running of the body. It:

- promotes flexible joints
- encourages good muscle tone
- supplies energy for working muscles
- provides an important structure/scaffold for the brain
- helps the body absorb vitamins and antioxidants
- helps to make vital hormones
- contributes to a healthy immune system
- maintains healthy skin and hair.

This list may not sound particularly important, and you may not immediately notice the benefits of including healthy oils in your diet. Yet the good sort of fats are crucial if a dancer wants to succeed as a performer.

You may recall from Chapter 2 that fat should provide around a quarter of your calorie intake, and, as fat contains over twice the calories compared with the same weight of carbohydrate and protein, the quantity of intake will feel less than this proportion.

It is the type of fat we eat that is particularly important, as each has a different purpose. 'Good' fats and 'bad' fats are terms often used to distinguish between fats that are important and fats that should be consumed in small quantities. Research shows that both dancers and general public eat too much saturated fat; so there is room for improvement.

Types of fat

The two types of fat in the diet are termed *saturated* and *unsaturated*. Unsaturated fats are divided into two groups, *monounsaturated* and *polyunsaturated*, and both are considered healthy choices. Saturated fats should be limited in the diet.

Monounsaturated – a first-rate fat

The best-known monounsaturated fat is olive oil, but rapeseed, groundnut, hazelnut and almond oils, olives, nuts and seeds are also good choices. Monounsaturated fats should provide around half of your total fat intake, and are considered to be the healthiest fats of all in terms of heart health.

> **Tip**
> To ensure you are getting the right amount of monounsaturated fat, for each person add a tablespoon of olive oil to salads, pasta dishes etc.

Polyunsaturated fat – the oil of choice

Most vegetable oils (such as sunflower oil) are good sources of polyunsaturated fats, and in small amounts these fats are an important part of the diet. Adding a tablespoon of vegetable oil in cooking will ensure that you are getting enough.

> **Tip**
> If you are adding a small amount of oil in cooking, avoid adding it again on the table, as you would then be doubling your intake.

The most important polyunsaturated fats, those at the top of a dancer's 'must include' list, are the omega oils. Including these polyunsaturated fats is key to a dancer's staying power. So what's their mission? They do the following:

- provide anti-inflammatory protection, preventing strains on joints, ligaments and tendons
- reduce inflammation associated with over-training
- promote healing of injuries
- improve delivery of oxygen and nutrients to cells
- increase stamina and energy levels.

The essential fats (known as omega-3 and omega-6) are found in oily fish such as mackerel, salmon, fresh tuna (not tinned), sardines, anchovies and kippers. Non-fish sources of essential fats include linseeds (flax seeds), linseed (flax) oil, pumpkin seeds, walnuts, rapeseed oil and soybeans. There is also a wide variety of foods fortified with essential fats that can be purchased in local food stores, such as omega-3 eggs, bread and fruit juice. One or two portions of oily fish each week, or one to three tablespoons of linseed oil, rapeseed oil, pumpkin seeds or walnuts each day, will guarantee that your diet provides sufficient amounts of the essential fats.

Which fats are known as bad fats?

Animal products are the main culprits containing high levels of unhealthy fats, and people who have high levels of saturated fat in their diet are also much more likely to be overweight or to struggle with their weight. Saturated fats do not contain more calories than other fats, but are associated with heart disease, stroke, high cholesterol and high blood pressure, and have no positive health benefits. Foods high in saturated fat include butter, lard, cheese, and the fat found in and around cuts of meat. Processed foods such as cakes, biscuits, pastries and other bakery products are also (unfortunately) high in saturated fat.

Fat is stored not only under the skin, but also between organs (heart, liver, kidneys) and within arteries. Too much fat stored beneath the skin (fat you can see) and too much fat within arteries and between organs is present in overweight individuals. However, before you conclude that you don't have a problem, normal-weight and even underweight people can also be at risk if they consume too much saturated fat. One can easily store fat within arteries and organs, and not under the skin where it can be more readily seen.

Why should I watch the amount of fat I have in my diet?

Dietary fat is the most energy dense of the three main nutrients. It has over twice the number of calories per gram as protein and carbohydrate do.

- 1g protein has 4 calories.
- 1g carbohydrate has 4 calories.
- 1g fat has 9 calories.

It is not necessarily the case that fat in the diet turns to fat within the body. Excessive amounts of any of the three main nutrients can lead to fat being stored in the body. Quite simply, extra calories are stored as fat, as that is how the body saves the energy it doesn't need straight away.

Tips for following a low fat diet

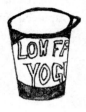 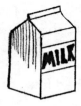 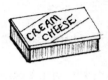

The tips in Table 4.1 will help you to follow a low-fat diet by substituting foods high in saturated fat with low-fat alternatives.

Table 4.1. Tips on following a low fat diet

Food group	Product	High-fat option	Low-fat alternative
Dairy products	Milk	Full-fat	Semi-skimmed or skimmed
	Yoghurt	Thick & creamy /Greek style yoghurt	Low-fat natural or fruit yoghurt, low-fat fromage frais
	Cheese	Full-fat hard or soft cheese	Reduced-fat cream cheese, half-fat hard cheese, cottage cheese
Red meat	Beef, lamb, pork, duck	Sausages, burgers, streaky bacon, spam, meat pies, fried meat.	Unprocessed meats, grilled red meat with visible fat removed, lean grilled bacon, low-fat sausages
Poultry	Chicken, turkey	Fried, breaded, battered, chicken with skin	Baked/grilled chicken without breadcrumbs, batter or skin. Lean chicken slices
Sauces	Sauces used in cooking	Cream or oil-based	Tomato based sauces, soy sauce, low-fat sauces
Cooking oils & spreads	Spreads	Butter, margarine, lard	Low-fat spread, olive-based spread
	Oils (vegetable oil, olive oil, animal fat)	Excessive amounts used in cooking and on the table	1 tablespoon of vegetable oil (if cooking), 1 tablespoon of olive oil (on salads or over dishes after being cooked)
Cakes, biscuits & pastries		Cream based, pastries, chocolate covered pastries.	English muffins, teacakes, scones (not butter varieties), home-made cakes and scones (see recipes)
Spreads		Butter, chocolate sauce, thick peanut butter spread	Low-fat cream cheese, honey, jam, marmalade, yeast extract, thin layer of peanut butter
Deserts		Ice cream, trifles	Sorbets, home-made trifles, jelly and fruit
Snacks		Chocolate/crisps/ chips	Cereal bars, snack-size chocolate bars, dried fruit bars

So what do we consider high fat, and what is considered healthy? To help you make a healthy choice, here is how to interpret and understand the nutritional information labels you find on food packages.

Amount of total fat
High fat (per 100g): More than 20g
Low fat (per 100g): 3g or less
(Medium level of fat is between these two values)

Amount of saturated fat (fats we should limit)
High fat (per 100g): More than 5g
Low fat (per 100g): 1.5g or less
(Medium level of fat is between these two values)

Is there a problem with following a very low-fat diet?

Very low-fat diets can lead to nutritional deficiencies and imbalances. The detrimental effects associated with such diets include:

- dull, flaky skin and other skin problems (e.g. eczema)
- cold extremities (fingers and toes) because the body is trying to preserve heat
- hormone imbalances and loss of menstruation
- poor control of inflammation and blood pressure
- lowered immune system and greater susceptibility to colds and viruses
- greater risk of injury
- slower recovery from injury
- inability to absorb important vitamins, including vitamins A, D and E
- greater risk of osteoporosis and brittle bones.

Chapter summary

- Fat is an essential part of every cell within the body, and plays a vital role in promoting flexible joints and good muscle tone, helping to fight off infections, and maintaining healthy skin and hair.

- Fat should contribute around 25 per cent of our daily calorie intake. To ensure you do not exceed this amount, where possible choose foods that are low in fat.
- Beneficial fats include fats that are unsaturated (monounsaturated and polyunsaturated).
- Monounsaturated fat should contribute around half of our total fat intake. Olive oil is a good source, as are nuts, seeds and rapeseed oil. In terms of heart health, these are considered to be the healthiest of all. Add a tablespoon of olive oil per person to salads or in cooking to ensure you are getting the right amount.
- Polyunsaturated fat is involved in many important functions in the body, including preventing joint, ligament and tendon strains, reducing inflammation and contributing to the healing of injuries. Good sources of polyunsaturated fat include most vegetable oils. The omega-3 and omega-6 polyunsaturated fats (which must be supplied by the diet, because the body is unable to make them) are found in oily fish such as salmon, mackerel, fresh tuna, sardines, anchovies and kippers, and in some vegetable sources such as linseed and soybeans. Include one or two portions of oily fish each week, or take a fish oil or flaxseed oil supplement with your diet.
- Saturated fats are considered unhealthy because they are associated with weight gain, heart disease and stroke. Saturated fats are predominately found in animal products such as meat and dairy produce. To limit saturated fat in your diet, simply choose low-fat dairy products and lean meat.

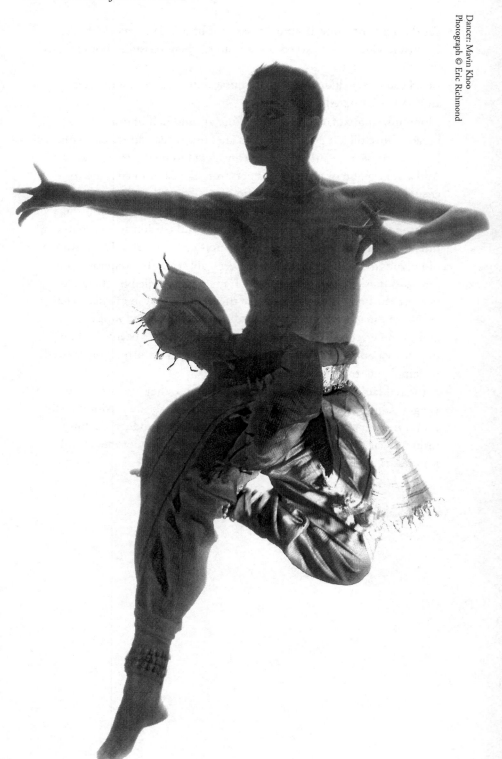

Chapter 5
Vitamins and Minerals

It takes an athlete to dance, but an artist to be a dancer.

Shanna La Fleur

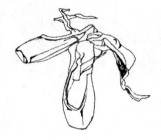

Imagine a tap shoe without the metal tap, classical ballet without the tutu, a performance without a curtain call, tango without the *paso básico*. The tiny crystals in a shimmering costume, the breadth in a dancer's leap can be the quintessential things that breathe life into dance: that *je ne sais quoi*.

Vitamins and minerals are found in minute quantities in the foods we eat; yet despite their size, vitamins and minerals are imperative to the dancer. Without them, the body's chemistry would just not work.

Vitamins

'Vita' is Latin for 'life'. In terms of dance, vitamins are an absolute necessity for vitality, strength, performance and expressing individuality. Although we require only very small amounts of each vitamin, many chemical activities within the body simply cannot occur unless the right vitamin is present. Some vitamins are attached to enzymes that can do their job only if the vitamin is part of the enzyme's structure. For example, vitamin B6 is part of an enzyme that is responsible for building new protein from amino acids, and the vitamin biotin is necessary for the enzyme responsible for breaking down fats. Other vitamins form part of the immune system, whilst others are involved in the nervous and hormone systems.

Most importantly, vitamins must be supplied by our diet, as our bodies are unable to make them.

There are two types of vitamin: *fat-soluble* and *water-soluble*. Fat-soluble vitamins (vitamin A, D, E and K) do not necessarily have to be included in the diet every day. In the case of a plentiful supply, the body can store excess amounts of these vitamins for future use. Water-soluble vitamins (B vitamins, vitamin C) must be included in the diet every day, because they are unable to be stored. Any extra is excreted in the urine.

Hint
Water-soluble vitamins are more vulnerable and are easily lost in cooking, as they leach out of the food into the water (you may notice the water turning a different colour after boiling vegetables).

Minerals

Minerals must be obtained from the foods we eat, because they cannot be made by the body.

Some minerals (such as calcium and phosphorus in bones and teeth) form part of structures within the body, while others are required for muscles to contract, or to control the fluid balance in tissues.

Important definitions

The **Recommended Daily Amount (RDA)** of a vitamin or mineral is the quantity that the Food Standards Agency advises that we should have each day to preserve our well-being. RDA is often quoted on the back of food packages.

The Reference Nutrient Intake (RNI) is the quantity sufficient for the daily nutrient needs for 97.5 per cent of the population.

Free radicals are small chemicals constantly produced by the body as a result of everyday lifestyle activities (digestion, breathing, walking, dancing). Free radicals are also produced when the body becomes exposed to environmental stress such as pollution, cigarette smoke or exhaust fumes. Once these substances are produced, the body needs to inactivate them, as free radicals can react and join to other substances within our body and produce chemicals that are damaging to the body. Damage from large quantities of free radicals is associated with cancer, heart disease, ageing and genetic abnormalities. In relation to dance, free-radical damage can lead to injury, muscle pain and fluid retention. The body works harder during dance and exercise, as it requires more oxygen and produces more heat, and muscles contract harder. The more you exercise, the more free radicals you make.

Antioxidants are enzymes and nutrients that help the body inactivate free radicals by changing the shape of the free radical and thus preventing it from being harmful. Many vitamins can be viewed as antioxidants, as they prevent damage caused by free radicals. Enzymes that act as antioxidants have minerals such as zinc, selenium and manganese incorporated into their structure. Thus one of the vital roles of vitamins and minerals is to protect the body against free-radical damage.

Vitamins and minerals important for the dancer

A full list of vitamins and minerals can be found in Appendix 6. In this section we look at the vitamins and minerals considered to be the most important for the dancer.

Vitamin C is especially important, as it is required for the growth and repair of tissues in all parts of the body. It is needed to form *collagen*, an important protein used to make skin, scar tissue, tendons, ligaments and blood vessels. Vitamin C is also vital for the healing of wounds, and for the repair and maintenance of cartilage, bones and teeth.

Vitamin C is a water-soluble vitamin needed in the diet every day, as it cannot be stored in the body. It is a powerful antioxidant, and has a further role by helping the body absorb iron from food.

> **Which foods contain Vitamin C?**
> All fruits and vegetables contain vitamin C. However, those having the greatest amount include citrus fruits, juices, strawberries, tomatoes, broccoli, sweet and white potatoes and cantaloupe.
>
>   Other excellent sources include papaya, mango, watermelon, Brussels sprouts, cauliflower, cabbage, winter squash, red peppers, raspberries, blueberries, cranberries and pineapples.

  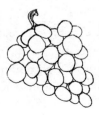

B vitamins are a collection of eight water-soluble vitamins that play a very important role in metabolism. Each B vitamin has a number and a name, and together they are often termed *vitamin B complex*:

B1 (thiamine)
B2 (riboflavin)
B3 (niacin)
B5 (pantothenic acid)
B6 (pyridoxine)
B7 (biotin)
B9 (folic acid)
B12 (cyanocobalamin)

The B vitamins work together to provide many health benefits to the dancer, such as supporting and increasing the rate of metabolism; breaking down carbohydrates, protein and fats from food; maintaining healthy skin and hair; and maintaining good muscle tone.

Which foods contain the B vitamins?
B vitamins come from a variety of natural sources, including potatoes, bananas, lentils, brewer's yeast, molasses and yeast extract. Many breakfast cereals and energy drinks are also fortified with them. Wholemeal breads and cereals contain more B vitamins than processed food products do.

Iron is a mineral found in every cell in the body. Most importantly for the dancer, iron helps the body make red blood cells, which transport oxygen to working muscles. Iron deficiency can lead to lack of energy, shortness of breath, headaches, dizziness, irritability and even hair loss. Dancers who are more likely to be iron deficient include those experiencing heavy periods, dancers who restrict their calorie intake, or those avoiding red meat.

Which foods contain iron?
Iron from animal sources is absorbed better than that from other sources, but it *is* possible to get enough iron from vegetable sources. Liver, red meat, beans, nuts, dried fruit (such as dried apricots), wholegrains (such as brown rice), fortified breakfast cereals, soybean flour and most dark green leafy vegetables (such as watercress and curly kale) are all good sources of iron. When combined with vitamin C (such as from fruit or fruit juice), iron absorption is maximised.

Calcium is the most plentiful mineral found in the human body and is also one of the most important. Teeth and bones contain the most calcium, with the rest found in nerve cells, body tissues and blood. Calcium helps muscles, including the heart, to contract and relax during dance and exercise, and reduces the risk of developing osteoporosis (thinning bones). Osteoporosis is alarmingly common in dancers and can hinder a promising career.

Which foods contain calcium?
Dairy products such as milk, yoghurt and cheese provide a great source of calcium. Low-fat dairy products contain the same amount of calcium as their full-fat counterparts, and are a much better choice. Two to four portions each day will guarantee a good supply of calcium (one portion is equivalent to a 150g pot of yoghurt, 200ml skimmed/semi-skimmed milk, 200ml soya milk fortified with calcium, or a matchbox-size portion of tofu or cheese).

Good vegetable sources include green leafy vegetables (such as broccoli and cabbage, but not spinach), soya beans, tofu, soya drinks with added calcium, nuts, bread and anything made with fortified flour. Fish with bones, such as sardines and pilchards, are also good sources of calcium. Soya products (such as milk and yoghurts) are a good source, but only if they are fortified, as soya does not contain calcium naturally.

Zinc is present in every part of the body and has many, many important functions for the dancer. Zinc helps the body produce new enzymes and cells, helps metabolise carbohydrates, fats and proteins in the food we eat, and also plays a very important role in maintaining a healthy immune system and healing wounds. Zinc is vital for the working of many of the body's systems, and is particularly important for healthy skin and resistance to infection. Zinc deficiency amongst dancers is relatively common.

Which foods contain zinc?
Zinc is found widely in foods, in which good sources include meat, shellfish and cereal products. Good vegetarian sources are dairy products, beans and lentils, yeast, nuts, seeds and wholegrain cereals. Pumpkin seeds provide one of the most concentrated plant sources of zinc.

Supplements – Do I need them and which ones are best?

If your diet is balanced and varied, and you are including all the food groups (see Table 3.1), then it is likely that you have a good intake of vitamins and minerals. However, in practice, many dancers do not plan their meals or snacks, or they restrict their calorie intake and avoid certain foods. If you travel a lot, work irregular hours or shifts and eat on the run, it can take considerably more effort to eat well, and so you run the risk of missing out on important nutrients.

If you feel your diet does not provide a healthy balance of nutrients, try to plan your meals and snacks to include more foods that are rich in vitamins and minerals. You may benefit from taking a multi-vitamin supplement if:

- you eat out a lot, or eat on the run
- you eat less than 1500 kcal a day
- you rely on processed foods
- you are a vegan (you may lack vitamin B12)
- you are anaemic (lack of iron)
- you are pregnant (you may lack folic acid)
- you are a heavy smoker/drinker.

Did you know?
Eating lots of processed food can rob your body of vitamins and minerals. To break down and get rid of unwanted chemicals in the food you have eaten, the body uses up valuable vitamins and minerals, thus depleting your stores.

Balance is the key

It is most definitely the *balance* of vitamins and minerals that is most important. An excess or deficiency of one vitamin could reduce the absorption of another; for example, a lack of vitamin C would reduce the absorption of iron. Healthy bones need a careful balance of vitamin D, calcium, phosphorus, magnesium, zinc manganese, fluoride, chloride, copper and boron! And although it is tempting to think that more is better, vitamins and minerals are required in certain amounts. An abundance will not continue to improve performance, nor will it increase the number of pirouettes you can do.

Unless advised otherwise by your doctor or nutritionist, it is best to take a multi-vitamin supplement, as imbalances and deficiencies are more likely to occur if you take a single vitamin or mineral supplement. With the exception of vitamin A from liver, it is very difficult to overdose on vitamins and minerals from food. However, certain vitamins and minerals can be quite harmful if excessive amounts are taken, so always follow the advice on the label or the advice of a dietitian or nutritionist (Appendix 6 gives advice on upper limits).

Exercise, vitamins and minerals

The RNI represents the nutrient needs of 97.5 per cent of the population, but dancers may have greater needs because of the amount of exercise they undertake during classes, rehearsals and performances. As you may remember, the harder the body works, the more free radicals are produced naturally. It makes sense, therefore, that more antioxidants in the form of vitamins and minerals are then needed to maintain the balance.

Tips

- Aim for five portions of fruit and vegetables each day.
- Choose fruits, vegetables and salads of different colours, as each colour indicates a different antioxidant or vitamin (dark green vegetables are rich in chlorophyll, tomatoes are rich in lycopene, carrots are rich in carotene).
- Add a side salad to your meals.
- Eat fresh fruit for a snack and/or dessert.

Summary

- Vitamins and minerals are found in minute quantities in the food we eat, and are vital for a dancer's health and performance.
- Vitamins must be supplied by the diet, because the body is unable to make them. Many vitamins are incorporated into the structure of enzymes, which cannot do their job if the vitamin is missing. As well as having other roles, enzymes promote a good metabolic rate and a healthy immune system.

- Many minerals contribute to structures within the body, such as teeth and bones. Like vitamins, they must be supplied by the diet. The most important minerals include calcium and iron.
- Processed foods can rob the body of vitamins and minerals, which we use to break down the artificial chemicals in processed foods and rid our bodies of them.
- Owing to busy lifestyles or a restricted intake, many dancers do not include optimal levels of both vitamins and minerals in their diet. Therefore including a multi-vitamin supplement, and planning nutrient-rich snacks and meals, can promote long-term health and improved performance.
- Some vitamins and minerals are toxic in high doses. Avoid taking a vitamin supplement that provides more than ten times the recommended nutrient intake (RNI). Taking individual vitamin and mineral supplements can also lead to imbalances and deficiencies, and so multi-vitamin supplements are preferable.

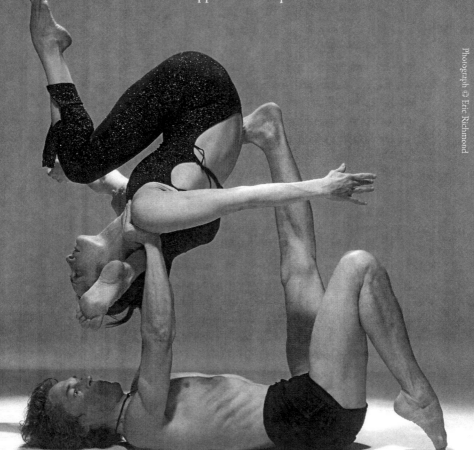

Photograph © Eric Richmond

Chapter 6
Fluid – The Fourth Macronutrient

The higher up you go, the more mistakes you are allowed.
Right at the top, if you make enough of them, it's considered
to be your style.

Fred Astaire

Water constitutes 70 per cent of the brain, 82 per cent of the blood and 90 per cent of the lungs. In fact, two-thirds of our entire body weight is water, and next to air it is the most essential substance for our survival. Despite its immense importance, however, water is often placed towards the bottom of a dancer's list of performance-enhancing nutrients.

Only in the presence of water can the body use stored fat for energy, move nutrients through the bloodstream, get rid of toxins that have accumulated and have resulted in fluid retention, allow enzyme reactions to occur (such as those involved in metabolism), and repair damaged tissues after injury. Our cells, tissues and organs all depend on water to function, and the reason it is often pushed to the bottom of the 'must have' pile is simple: the less you drink, the less able your body is to recognise when it is dehydrated.

Losing fluid during dance

Extra heat produced during dance must be lost to the environment to ensure that our body temperature does not exceed 36.5°C. To do this, fluid is lost through sweat and through water vapour in the air we breathe out. Water from the body is carried to the skin, and as it evaporates, our bodies lose heat. A dancer can lose as much as 2 litres of water in a single rehearsal or performance.

Heat, you may recall, is a form of energy, and therefore losing heat means you are burning energy and using up calories.

The amount of sweat you produce, or the amount of water lost through your skin, depends on how hard you are dancing, how long you are dancing for, the temperature of the room and your individual body chemistry (some people naturally sweat less or more than others). On average you lose around 600kcal of heat energy for every litre of sweat.

Tip
To measure approximately how much fluid is lost during a class or performance, weigh yourself before and after. Every 1kg reduction in body weight represents 1 litre of fluid.

Consequences of dehydration

Even losing 2 per cent of your weight in fluid can have a dramatic effect not only on your performance, but also on your health. As blood is predominantly made up of water, dehydration decreases the volume of your blood and makes it more concentrated. As your body temperature rises during exercise, extra stress is placed on the heart and lungs, and your heart has to work extra hard to pump blood around your body and deliver oxygen to your muscles. This means that exercise becomes much harder and your performance levels become sluggish. The more dehydrated you become, the less able your body is to sweat, meaning that your body temperature rises and your health is put at risk.

When your body becomes dehydrated, you also run the risk of developing a sluggish metabolic rate (water is needed for healthy digestion), and are more likely to hold excess body fat and retain water. Poor muscle tone, joint and muscle soreness and cramps are all associated with poor fluid intake and dehydration.

How will I know if I am dehydrated?

When you dance, it is natural and desirable to sweat, as it is the body's way of regulating body temperature. When you become dehydrated, you may experience symptoms of general tiredness, sluggishness and headaches, and feel light-headed or nauseous. A very accurate (though admittedly not very glamorous) way of monitoring your fluid status is to observe the colour intensity of your urine. Pale yellow indicates that you have the right hydration status: dark yellow means you are dehydrated.

> **Hint**
> If you feel thirsty, you are already dehydrated! What's more, the body is not always very good at telling you when it's dehydrated. Sometimes when you are feeling hungry, it's actually your body's way of saying it's thirsty.

Your average daily fluid requirements

Experts suggest that the average adult requires around 2 litres of fluid intake (approximately 8 glasses) per day, of which at least half should come from water. Dancers require slightly more than this because they lose fluid during exercise. If you become dehydrated, the good thing is that you can correct it immediately by consuming fluid in the form of water or juice.

Preventing dehydration before, during and after dance

If you begin to exercise in a dehydrated state, your performance is naturally going to suffer and become more and more sluggish as you continue to practise. The best way to prevent dehydration is to start a class or performance in a hydrated state.

Before exercise

The more fluid you have in your stomach, the more quickly it gets absorbed. So try to drink most of your fluid needs for exercise at the beginning of your class or performance. The British Dietetic Association suggests drinking around 400–600ml of fluid 2 hours before exercise, which allows time for your body to absorb enough fluid (and also allows for that rather annoying but all-important trip to the bathroom!).

During a dance class or performance

The more you sweat, the more fluid you will need to replace it; but, for guidance, aim for 150–350ml every 20 minutes (depending on how intense your training is). *Do not* wait until you feel thirsty, and *do not* try to drink all your requirements at the end! *Do* go by how you feel, and drink as much as you feel comfortable with.

Wearing several layers of clothing (particularly synthetic fibres that promote sweating) and dancing in very warm environmental conditions can make a dancer much more prone to dehydration. In these situations, try to stay as hydrated as possible by drinking small amounts of fluid regularly.

> **Tip**
> You may find that you are able to drink more if the fluid is more palatable and in a container that makes drinking easy. Try to keep your drinks cool (15–22°C) and choose one for which you find it easy to drink the quantity you need.

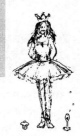

After dance

Immediately after dance, you must replace the fluid lost. Drinking before and during exercise will really help you to keep hydrated, and on average, a dancer will need to drink around 1.5 litres of fluid after exercise to replenish fluid lost through sweat.

I can't drink that much! It makes me feel bloated/nauseous

If you feel nauseous or experience any discomfort (such as bloating, cramps, discomfort or heaviness) when you drink water or any other type of drink, it could mean you are dehydrated. Even a small amount of dehydration slows down digestion and the rate at which your stomach empties, leading to feelings of bloatedness, cramps and nausea. Discomfort could also be caused by drinking fluids high in sugar, as concentrated drinks take longer to empty from the stomach than do more dilute drinks.

If you think you could be dehydrated, try to drink as much as you comfortably can before dancing, even if this means starting with small sips. Then continue to drink small amounts during the class or performance. If you think the sugar-based drinks you are choosing are causing discomfort, dilute them further by adding more water. It is all about finding what works best for you, and a little trial and error may be all it takes to strike a comfortable balance.

Types of fluid

Table 6.1 recommends the kind of drink to consider taking, depending on the degree of exercise you undertake.

Table 6.1. Which drink?

Exercise time & intensity	Drink
Less than 30 minutes	Water
Low to moderate intensity, less than 1 hour	Water
Moderate to high intensity, less than 1 hour	Water or hypotonic drink
High intensity, more than 1 hour	Hypotonic or isotonic drink

Hypotonic drinks aim to replace fluid rather than provide energy. They contain a certain amount of carbohydrates and electrolytes that make the body absorb fluid faster than it would water. On average, a hypotonic drink contains around 4g carbohydrate per 100ml. It can be made with diluted fruit juice or fruit squash (see Appendix 1 for recipes).

    Isotonic drinks contain more carbohydrate than hypotonic drinks do, and are absorbed at about the same rate as water. Isotonic drinks are therefore used to replace fluid *and* provide energy. They too can be made from diluted fruit juice and fruit squash. On average, they should contain 4–8g carbohydrate per 100ml (see Appendix 1 for recipes).

Other non-alcoholic drinks

Diet drinks or 'sugar-free' drinks contain artificial sweeteners, which have not been shown to have any positive or negative effect on performance. They contain very little carbohydrate, but can help replace fluid at around the same rate as water. If you find it difficult to drink just water and prefer to drink something flavoured, choose these types of drinks (e.g. for low- to moderate-intensity exercise lasting less than 1 hour).

    Carbonated drinks hydrate the body equally as well as still drinks. However, some people experience mild heartburn, stomach discomfort or a feeling of fullness. You may prefer lightly carbonated drinks, but it is down to individual preference. Do be aware, however, that consuming fizzy drinks in excess may increase the risk of developing osteoporosis because of their phosphorus content (see Chapter 11).

Caffeinated drinks such as coffee, tea, cola and some sports drinks contain caffeine, a stimulant that can increase alertness and improve performance. Some sports drinks also contain extract of guarana – a plant that contains caffeine. A moderate intake of caffeine will not dehydrate the body for those who drink it regularly (equivalent to three cups of coffee per day). Caffeine in large doses, or when taken by individuals who may be more sensitive to caffeine, can have a diuretic effect by increasing water excretion (urination). Some people also experience other symptoms such as shaking, rapid heartbeat and anxiety.

Alcohol

On days where you do not train, drinking alcohol within sensible limits is perfectly acceptable. However, drinking alcohol before exercise, even in small amounts, can have unwanted effects, such as:

- reducing speed and strength
- lowering blood sugar levels
- increasing the risk of dehydration caused by increased water excretion (urination)
- increasing the risk of injury
- reducing balance, coordination and precision.

Alcohol and calories – can alcohol make me gain weight?

Alcohol contains 7kcal per gram – more than protein and carbohydrate, but less than fat. Any food or drink, including alcohol, can encourage weight gain if you exceed your calorie requirements; therefore you *can* gain weight if you take in excess calories through alcohol.

Summary

- Our cells, tissues, and organs all depend on fluid and cannot function without it. Only with sufficient water can the body use fat for energy, repair damaged muscle cells and promote a good metabolic rate.

- Dehydration has a dramatic effect on performance, making the dancer likely to suffer from fatigue, aching muscles, cramps, sluggishness, headaches and dizziness. Other effects of dehydration include reduced digestion time, excess body fat, poor muscle tone and water retention.
- A very accurate way to measure your hydration is to observe the colour of your urine: dark yellow means you are dehydrated, pale yellow means you are well hydrated.
- Experts suggest that we need around 2 litres of fluid intake each day, of which at least half should come from water. Dancers may need more because of fluid losses during exercise and performance in warm environments.
- Aim to drink around 400–600ml of fluid up to 2 hours before dancing (2–3 glasses). This allows time for your body to absorb enough fluid, and for you to have a trip to the bathroom!
- Aim to drink 150–300ml every 20 minutes whilst dancing (depending on how intense your training is).
- After dancing, drink as much as comfortably possible so that you are not dehydrated for your next dance session.
- If you are thirsty, you are already dehydrated!
- Your choice of fluid will depend on how much you need and what you prefer to drink. Choose between water, a hypotonic drink (which replaces fluid more quickly than water does) and an isotonic drink (which is absorbed at about the same rate as water, but also provides energy).
- Fluids are more palatable when they are cool and in a container that makes drinking easy.
- Diet drinks are absorbed at the same rate as water. If you find it difficult to drink enough water, choose these types of drinks.
- Caffeinated drinks can lead to dehydration if too much is consumed, or if you are sensitive to the effects of caffeine (increased urination, rapid heartbeat and anxiety). A moderate amount of caffeine (equivalent to three cups of coffee per day) can increase alertness and improve performance.
- On days when you train, it is advisable to avoid alcohol. On days where you do not train, drinking within safe limits is acceptable.

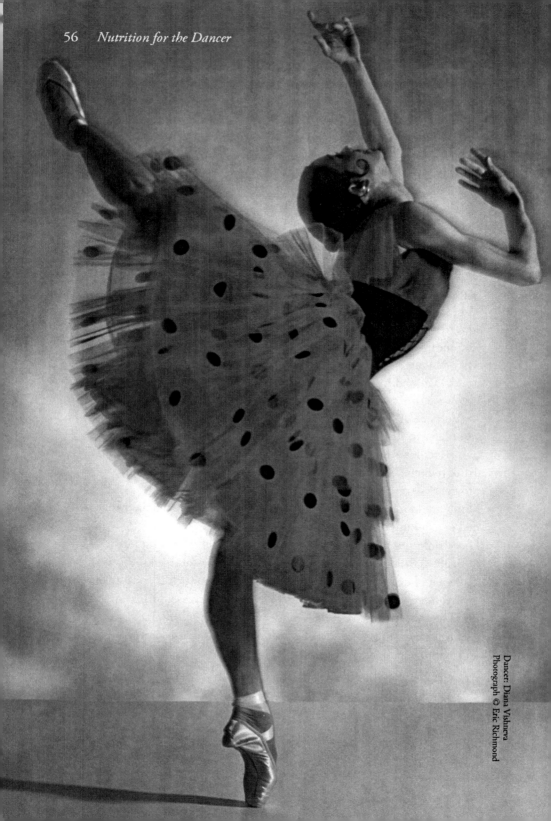

Interlude

The Dancer on the Road

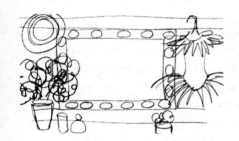

I have performed for thousands when they found me exotic, the vogue, daring, but I have danced, at any given time, for about ten people ... They were the ones that left the theatre forever different from the way they were when they came in. All of my long, long life, I have danced for those ten.

Ruth St. Denis

Touring with a dance company is likely to involve overseas travelling, different time zones, long and tedious spells of waiting, coach journeys, trains and even the odd boat. You may find each stop lasts only a few days, and then you are back on the road towards another city and another time zone. Such a jet-setting dancer's life will unfortunately have its consequences: travel sickness, a woozy head, sleeplessness and that unbelievable alcohol-free hangover feeling. This will no doubt creep into and have an unwanted effect on your energy, your *joie de vivre* and, ultimately, your stage performance. Yet it doesn't stop there: eating unfamiliar foods and trying to find snacks and meals that will help you to perform well just add to the pressure of touring.

The following tips are specifically aimed at the frazzled dancer to help minimise touring woes so that you can concentrate on the purpose of your travel: your stage and its awaiting audience.

On the road

Ginger is a gem for overcoming travel sickness. If you suffer from nausea and queasiness, sipping a cup of ginger tea, sucking some ginger lozenges or taking a ginger capsule (500mg three times a day) will most certainly take the edge off, or dispel sickness completely.

For a little sleep on the journey, sprinkle a few drops of lavender or camomile essential oils on a cotton handkerchief or pillow. Take slow, deliberate breaths and allow the tension in your muscles to ease gradually.

Avoid alcohol, and limit caffeine to an occasional milky coffee or tea if you are trying to regulate your body. Alternatively, for a quick fix, a coffee with a double espresso hit should go down rather well.

On finally arriving at your destination, don't be tempted to try to stay awake for as long as physically possible (without enlisting a friend to sing or blow in your ear). A relaxing soak in a bath with a few drops of lavender and grapefruit essential oil will ease tension from your stressed muscles – enough to promote sleep for a few hours.

Try to eat light, familiar foods rather than rich, heavy, sauce-based dishes, particularly if your body thinks breakfast now consists of a heavy meal. Spicy, chilli and fatty dishes are not exactly helpful to the suffering dancer. Go for the bland (but very sensible) local delicacy and you won't regret your choice.

Protein-rich foods, vegetables and fruit can energise a sluggish body that has yet to catch up with a different time zone.

Pasta, rice and other starchy foods can help to settle jumpy nerves.

Sleepless nights

Lack of sleep can become quite a debilitating problem when you're asking your body to perform night after night. Insufficient hours of sleep may leave you feeling shattered and stressed, and concentration will most certainly waver on stage. A vicious cycle will form, preventing you from sleeping properly on consecutive nights.

Sleep triggers the release of growth hormones that help your body cells to absorb nutrients, feed the repair and growth of muscle and bone and, very importantly, boost your immune system. So sleep is vital for the dancer – and you need good quality sleep: deep sleep.

Avoid sweet foods such as biscuits, cakes and chocolate. They will make your blood sugars rise and promote grand *jetés* across the room. Cheese and meat = nightmares.

Starch stimulates the body to produce serotonin, a hormone that makes you feel very content. So make yourself a bowl of pasta, or a bowl of porridge with cow's milk, soya or rice milk, to induce sleep.

A glass of warm milk: old-fashioned admittedly, but it still works! Milk contains substances that kick-start the brain to produce serotonin. Just don't add cocoa: caffeine will reverse the effect.

> **Tip**
> Although going to bed with hunger pangs certainly won't contribute
> to restful and contented sleep, retiring on a full stomach could spell
> indigestion and fretful sleep. So avoid eating too late and too much;
> leave around 2 hours between a starchy meal and your duvet.

Herbal help: camomile, lemon balm, passion flower and valerian can lull
you into the perfect slumber. Sandalwood or marjoram essential oils in the bath
can also ease away tense muscles and stresses.

General tiredness

Have smaller, more frequent meals to keep blood sugars from rising and
dipping, and avoid anything too sugary.

Drink plenty of fluid in the form of water, herbal tea, fruit teas and low-
sugar squashes (alcohol and caffeine can result in energy highs and lows). You
might be pleasantly surprised to learn that your fatigue was down to
dehydration, and the results will be instant. Lemon tea can awaken a burnt-
out body.

Include plenty of fresh fruit, vegetables and wholegrain cereals: they are
bursting with B vitamins, which boost energy levels and a general feeling of
wellness.

Spirulina is a blue-green algae naturally very rich in highly digestible
nutrients. It is one of the most concentrated foods known, containing nine
important vitamins and over fourteen minerals that the body can absorb
extremely well – a great natural energy booster!

> **Note**
> If you are completely exhausted over an extended period of time,
> I suggest a brief visit to your doctor for a simple blood test, as tiredness
> could be a sign of several different health issues, such as anaemia or
> a hormone imbalance.

Colds and flu

A sore throat, a pounding head and an aching body in the shape of the common,
annoying cold is not always something you can avoid: air conditioning,

enclosed environments and frequent travel will expose you to a host of familiar and unfamiliar bacteria and viruses. Intense exercise can also suppress the immune system, and dancers can be very susceptible to upper respiratory tract infections, making the mouth and throat especially vulnerable.

The problem with over-the-counter remedies is that, while they may alleviate the symptoms at the time, they may do virtually nothing to boost your immune system, meaning that you are just as vulnerable to those little beasties as before. The very best results mean fighting off the cold whilst strengthening your immune system. You may not be able to avoid every cold milling around, but you can control how quickly you ward them off and, even better, build up your defences to keep them away.

Vitamin C	☑ Improve recovery	☑ Keep colds at bay

Vitamin C tops the list of great immune boosters: it occurs naturally in many fruits and vegetables, and supplements are relatively inexpensive. Include at least six servings of fruit and vegetables each day. If you decide to take a vitamin supplement, choose a multi-vitamin, and avoid taking more than 1000mg per day.

Zinc	☑ Improve recovery	☑ Keep colds at bay

Zinc is a very important mineral with great immune-system-boosting properties. Dancers tend to be deficient in this mineral, so you can make sure you're getting enough by including meat, shellfish and cereal products in your diet. Good vegetarian sources include dairy products, beans and lentils, yeast, nuts, seeds and wholegrain cereals. Pumpkin seeds provide one of the most concentrated plant sources of zinc.

Fluid, fluid, and a little more fluid will certainly help your body flush away toxins and clear congestion. Aim to drink at least 1.5–2 litres each day (8 glasses)

Dairy products have still not been proven scientifically to increase mucus production, but if you notice that for you they have a negative effect, cut back on them, remembering to replace dairy with other sources of the vital mineral calcium (fortified soya products, small-boned fish such as sardines, dried fruit and seeds).

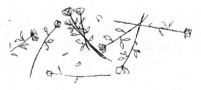

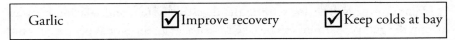

| Garlic | ☑ Improve recovery | ☑ Keep colds at bay |

Garlic is a member of the onion family, and has both antiseptic and decongestant properties, amongst many other powerful health benefits. Similarly to vitamin C and zinc, garlic also stimulates the multiplication of white blood cells, which play a leading role in fighting infections.

Concoctions
1 medium garlic clove crushed with a piece of root ginger of the same size. Mix this with 1 lemon and 1 teaspoon of honey. Add warm water and drink up to three cups each day.

If garlic doesn't exactly appeal to the taste buds (or your friends), mix lemon juice with 1 teaspoon of honey and ½ teaspoon of cinnamon powder.

| Echinacea | ☑ Improve recovery | ☑ Keep colds at bay |

Herbal help: Echinacea is one of the oldest and most popular herbal remedies to help fight infections. Unlike antibiotics that kill bacteria, echinacea indirectly fights infections by strengthening the body's immune system.

Heartburn and indigestion

These two afflictions can be quite painful and completely incapacitating. Erratic eating patterns, daily stresses and a bombardment of rich, heavy food can leave your body howling for respite. And you will soon know when it does ...

If you are prone to indigestion or heartburn, certainly avoid acidic foods such as vinegar and pickles, and stay away from fatty foods such as crisps, chips, nuts and fried or creamy dishes. Other food culprits inducing discomfort include some raw vegetables – onions, peppers, chillies, garlic – and some fruits, particularly citrus and unripe fruits.

Try to create a 'space' around a meal. Take time out to relax 5 or 10 minutes before and after a meal: take your time, eat slowly and not too much at once. Other tips such as not drinking too much whilst eating can also help. Cut down on alcohol and caffeine. Smoking is also an offender.

If indigestion persists, some instances of indigestion could be due to bacteria in the digestive system, so it might be worth a visit to your doctor, and possibly a course of antibiotics.

Peppermint is great for settling the digestive system and relaxing muscles within the gut. Peppermint can be taken as a tea, as lozenges or as peppermint oil.

Eating on the go, takeaways and fast foods, and restaurant dining

This section is for dancers who frequently find themselves having to buy a meal at a roadside shop or have trouble finding tasty and healthy food when on tour and on the road, dancers who want to eat out with friends, and dancers who have no or very little time to prepare a meal at home.

Eating on the go

One of the best ways of ensuring you always have something nutritious to snack on is to plan ahead and carry plenty of snacks. These can include packets of dried fruit, nuts and seeds, muesli cereal bars, crispbreads, fruit, salad sticks, mini pitta breads, English muffins, Scotch pancakes, scones, crumpets, potato cakes and teacakes. Second best is to choose the best options in the store where you are shopping. Table I.1 gives a few pointers.

Table I.1. Eating on the go

Food	Choose this ...
Light bites	Oat cereal bars, dried fruit bars, individually wrapped fruit-based biscuits, garibaldi biscuits

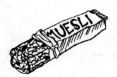

... instead of this
Chocolate, sweets, cakes.

Choose this ...

Sandwiches, wraps, rolls, baguettes, pitta bread, bagel, jacket potato	Fillings: chicken pieces/slices, tuna, salmon, ham slices and salad, light cream cheese, cottage cheese. Tomato-based dressings

... instead of this
Cheese/tuna and mayonnaise fillings, processed meat (spam, pâté, bacon).

Food	Choose this ...
Burgers and fast foods	Grilled chicken burger, vegetable burger, fish burger, plain chicken kebab with salad (no creamy dressings). Tomato-based sauce and salad and/or baked beans
	... instead of this
	Beef burger and chips, chicken batter/breadcrumbs, burgers with cheese, hot dogs, battered fish and chips, mayonnaise.
	Choose this ...
High-energy snacks	Flapjacks, sesame snaps, peanut butter sandwiches
	... instead of this
	Sausage rolls, pork pies, all meat, cheese and vegetables in pastry.

Takeaways and fast foods

Table I.2. Takeaways and fast foods

Food	The good ...
Japanese food	Rice noodles, soup, vegetables and stir-fries
	... the bad and the ugly
	Raw fish and rice can harbour food-poisoning bacteria, so tread carefully and watch for cleanliness in the restaurant.
	The good ...
Thai food	Soups, chillies, lemon grass, non-dairy foods and noodle-based dishes. Chicken seafood and vegetable dishes, plain rice
	... the bad and the ugly
	Prawn crackers, coconut curries, fatty meat dishes, fried rice. Green curries and chilli may prove problematic if you have a tendency to suffer from heartburn.

Food	**The good ...**
Kebabs	Chicken and lean lamb doner kebabs can be healthy choices when accompanied with plenty of salad and without dressings

... the bad and the ugly

Fatty meats, fatty creamy dressings, and lots of it.

The good ...

Pizzas More base, less cheese, and toppings such as chicken, fish, vegetables with a side salad

... the bad and the ugly

4 cheeses, thin crispy base, pepperoni, sausage, bacon, lots of cheese and a side-order of chips. Bad ... but sounds good.

The good ...

Jacket potatoes Tuna in a tomato-based sauce or light cream cheese, baked beans, lean mince in tomato sauce, chicken pieces, quorn pieces, tofu

... the bad and the ugly

Cheese, mayonnaise, butter, bacon and fatty meats.

Eating in restaurants

If you choose the right dishes, eating out with friends can be just as healthy and low in fat as when you prepare your own meals at home. Here are a few suggestions.

1. Aim to have just one starch portion with the meal (unless you have had a particularly demanding performance and need plenty of carbohydrate). This could be either the crusty bread served before the meal (without the butter) or the potatoes, rice, pasta or any other starchy food with your main course. Alternatively, you can have two smaller portions of both, such as a small amount of crusty bread beforehand and a small amount of carbohydrate with the main meal.

2. Try to avoid crisps, nuts and other fatty tasties on the table before your meal. Instead opt for a herbal tea, water or a spicy tomato juice, for instance.

3. Choose light dishes such as grilled chicken, fish or meat cooked in a tomato sauce or light fresh stock rather than copious amounts of creamy thick sauces and fatty meats.

4. Order salads and plenty of vegetables as part of the meal or as a side serving. Avoid creamy high-fat dressings, and ask for the dressing to be served separately or on the side so that you can add the amount you want.

5. Desserts can range from quite calorific pastries and pies, to light fruit-based desserts and fresh fruit. Opt for sorbets and yoghurt-based fruit desserts rather than pies and pastries.

6. Round off a meal with a good-quality coffee or a herbal/fruit tea. If you are performing the next day, it is best to stay clear of alcohol. If you are not on stage the following day, keep to small quantities and drink with water.

7. If the restaurant does not look clean, and the food does not look particularly appetising, do not risk it, as otherwise you may walk out with a few nasties in your digestive system!

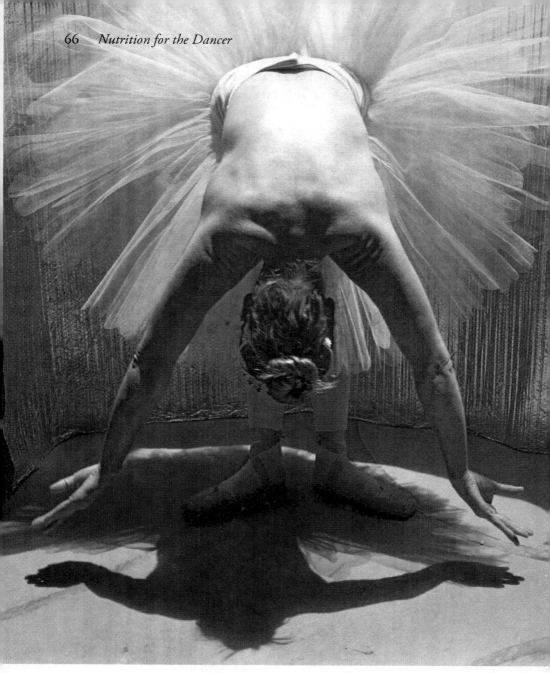

Photograph © Kim Weston

Part 2

Nutrition's Dance with the Body

The one important thing I have learnt over the years is the difference between taking one's work seriously and taking oneself seriously. The first is imperative and the second disastrous.

Dame Margot Fonteyn

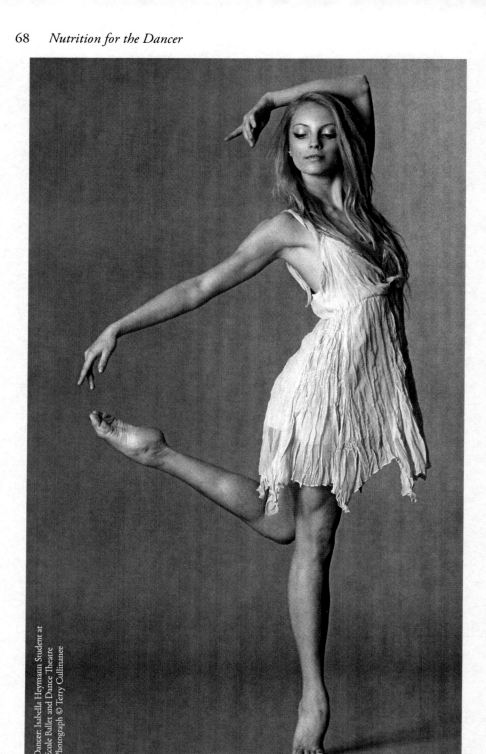

Chapter 7
The Young Dancer

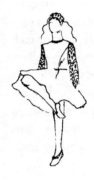

Young dancers are training at a very vulnerable time in their lives ... So train the whole person, not just the dancer.

Deborah Bull

Becoming a highly skilled dancer, or aspiring to a career on stage, demands many, many years of dedicated practice. Each objective accomplished, whether an extra pirouette, a difficult balance or a new grade passed, builds upon the skills previously mastered – an ever-growing tree of expertise and skill.

This is precisely how I view the young developing body.

Growing muscles, strong bones, flexible and supple joints need good nutrition. It is what shapes a dancer's future. And feeding the growing body must be given as much importance as a new step or another exam. During this period of training, the young dancer will develop their skill – the tool to their art.

Food and eating is a joy, a pastime that brings families, friends and new acquaintances closer together: laughter, jokes, old tales and storytelling all take place over the dining table. I cannot stress how fundamentally important it is for the young dancer to have a healthy attitude towards food – not just in terms of their growing body, but for their lifelong association with food. The matter of body shape is guaranteed to become a subject that a young dancer will be faced with, time and time again, at various points in their career. Confidence in body shape and food choices should be with them always, and building these relationships at an early stage is priceless. This cannot be stressed enough. Having a healthy, lean body means having a healthy attitude to food.

Some young dancers may struggle to keep up their weight, whilst others may be trying to keep trim. This chapter deals with key information for parents and teachers on the nutritional needs of young dancers, the importance of particular nutrients, and ways to help manage these issues.

Energy needs

There are two reasons why the energy needs of a young dancer are higher than those of a mature dancer (in terms of calories per kilogram of body weight): their bodies are maturing and growing, and they do not move as efficiently (they 'waste' energy compared with adults doing the same activity, as they lack coordination and make more movements because of inexperience).

Appendix 2 focuses on the recommended balance of foods in a diet appropriate for people over the age of 5 years. There are no specific data on children and young adults who exercise regularly, and it is rather difficult to predict exactly how much they need. For those individuals of an ideal weight, appetite and energy levels can be used to estimate portion sizes and whether they are eating enough.

The growing dancer and protein

Young dancers should try to include two to four portions of protein-rich foods each day (lean meat, fish, poultry, eggs, dairy products, beans, nuts, tofu and quorn). Their requirements are slightly higher than those of children or teenagers who do not exercise, at around 1.1–1.2g per kg of bodyweight per day. As with mature dancers, protein contributes around 15–20 per cent of other total energy needs.

Table 7.1. Nutritional intake for males (per day)

Age	Energy (EAR)*	Protein	Iron	Zinc	Salt
1–3yrs	1230 kcal	15g	7mg	5mg	2.2g
4–6yrs	1715 kcal	20g	6mg	6.5mg	3g
7–10yrs	1970 kcal	28g	9mg	7mg	5g
11–14yrs	2220 kcal	42g	11mg	9mg	6g
15–18yrs	2755 kcal	55g	11mg	9.5mg	6g

* Estimated average requirements

Table 7.2. Nutritional intake for females (per day)

Age	Energy (EAR)*	Protein	Iron	Zinc	Salt
1–3yrs	1165 kcal	15g	7mg	5mg	2.2g
4–6yrs	1545 kcal	20g	6mg	6.5mg	3g
7–10yrs	1740 kcal	28g	9mg	7mg	5g
11–14yrs	1845 kcal	41g	15mg	9mg	6g
15–18yrs	2110 kcal	45g	15mg	7mg	6g

* Estimated average requirements

Source (tables 7.1 and 7.2): *Dietary reference values for food energy and nutrients for the United Kingdom.* Report on Health and Social Subjects. Department of Health. London HMSO (1991).

Crown copyright material is reproduced with the permission of the Controller of Her Majesty's Stationery Office.

Carbohydrate

Carbohydrate supplies around 50 per cent of a young dancer's diet. Not only will carbohydrate be used to fuel their dancing, but it will 'save' protein so that it is used for growth instead of being broken down for energy to dance. To get the right balance of nutrients, base a meal or snack around a healthy source of carbohydrate, then decide on the source of protein.

Fat

Children and young adults need extra calories and nutrients to support them while they are growing. However, to maintain good health and general fitness, they need to ensure that their diet is balanced, and that means eating small amounts of healthy fats and limiting saturated unhealthy fats. For young dancers who are underweight or overweight, see the full discussion later in this chapter. Chapter 4 also explains which fats are considered healthy and which unhealthy.

Healthy meals and snacks

The following meal and snack ideas have a good balance of carbohydrate and protein, and just a little fat. The precise portion size depends on the individual's energy needs: bigger portions will be needed for older and more active children and teenagers, though you should be guided by their appetite, energy levels and weight.

Healthy meals for the young dancer (breakfast/lunch/dinner)

2–3 hours before training, with a drink of water.

- Healthy breakfast cereal with semi-skimmed milk and a banana
- Porridge with raisins and a teaspoon of honey
- Sandwich/roll/bagel/wrap/pitta filled with tuna, chicken, peanut butter or jam
- Jacket potato with tuna, chicken, baked beans or small amount of cheese
- Pasta with tomato-based sauce and lean mince (meat or quorn)
- Rice or noodles with chicken or fish
- Homemade vegetable stew.

Healthy snacks

1 hour before exercise, with a drink of water:

- Fresh fruit and a glass of semi-skimmed milk
- Home-made muffins and cakes (see recipes) or mini-bagels, mini-pancakes
- Handful of dried fruit
- Handful of dried fruit and nuts
- Healthy cereal bar or dried fruit bar
- Small wholemeal sandwich with jam, hummus or individual cheese portions
- Pot of yoghurt and a piece of fruit
- Flavoured milk or yoghurt drink
- Bowl of healthy cereal with semi-skimmed milk
- Wholemeal crackers or crispbread with cream cheese or chicken slices
- Plain popcorn.

Eating before a class/audition

Foods eaten before a class, a performance or an audition need to provide enough fuel to prevent lapses in energy levels. It must also be easily digested and familiar; so avoid offering anything new before an important audition or performance, as it may not agree with the young dancer. High-sugar snacks and drinks should also be avoided just before exercise, as they may cause a large increase in blood sugars followed by a rapid fall. Such fluctuations in blood sugars could result in early fatigue and also contribute to anxiety and bouts of nervous energy! The snack ideas provided above will prevent young dancers feeling hungry during exercise, will keep them going during the class, are easily digested, and do not cause a rapid increase in blood sugars.

Tips on food choices before an important event

- Choose familiar foods and drinks.
- Before the event, decide on suitable portion sizes by trial and error.
- Take your own food where possible.
- If the dancer is nervous, encourage them to have something light but nutritious, such as a milk based drink, a small yoghurt or yoghurt drink, diluted fruit juice or a light snack.
- Try not to skip meals, as young dancers may become light-headed or nauseous, and will not perform at their best.
- Choose snacks high in carbohydrate to provide enough fuel for working muscles.
- Avoid foods high in fat.
- Avoid eating sugary sweets.
- Avoid sugary drinks.
- Visit the bathroom just before the event!

Eating between classes or rehearsals

A water bottle for regular drink breaks is sufficient if exercise lasts 90 minutes or less. If lessons or rehearsals take place throughout a full day, try to take a supply of snacks and light meals high in carbohydrate to keep energy levels high. Portable, quick and easy-to-eat snacks are listed overleaf:

Healthy snacks, during training or rehearsal breaks

- Diluted fruit juice, milk/yoghurt drinks, water
- Fresh fruit – apples, pears, bananas, grapes, satsumas
- Dried fruit
- Cereal, energy and fruit bars
- Crispbread, crackers or rice cakes with jam, banana or peanut butter
- Rolls, sandwiches, mini-bagels, Scotch pancakes, English muffins.

Eating after a class or an audition

Young dancers are likely to be dehydrated after exercise, so the immediate priority is to replenish lost fluid with water or diluted fruit juice. If more than half an hour elapses between exercise and a main meal, choose a healthy 'recovery snack' to keep hunger at bay and help recovery. Eating as soon as possible after exercise is very important, as it dictates how quickly and effectively a young dancer recovers before the next class or performance.

The lists below provide ideas on suitable recovery snacks and meals. They contain a moderate amount of sugar (for quick recovery and storage in muscle) and also protein, which has also been shown to enhance recovery further.

Try to avoid snacks such as chocolate bars, crisps, sweets, pastries and fizzy drinks, as they do not promote good recovery after exercise. Not only do they contain high levels of calories in the form of sugar and fat, they are 'empty' calories, as these items are low in the vitamins and minerals that healthier foods have in abundance.

Healthy snacks after exercise

- Fresh fruit – apples, pears, bananas, grapes
- Smoothies
- Fruit yoghurt or yoghurt drink
- Dried fruit, nuts and raisins
- Home-made muffin, biscuits (see recipes)
- Cereal bar or fruit bar.

Healthy meals after exercise

Include one or two portions of vegetables or salad, and a glass of water.

- Pasta in tomato sauce with chicken, tuna, lean red meat or quorn
- Rice with chicken and vegetables/salad
- Jacket potato with beans, tuna or lean mince in tomato sauce
- Potato and fish pie (see recipe)
- Bean/Quorn burger with a wholemeal bap
- Baked beans on toast
- Tuna or chicken sandwich with lettuce and tomato.

The young dancer and the risk of dehydration

Young dancers are more vulnerable than adults to dehydration, because they often fail to recognise feelings of thirst, are more likely to overheat, and sweat less. How much fluid they lose during exercise depends on how long they exercise for, the intensity of exercise, their size (the bigger they are, the greater the fluid loss) and their fitness (the fitter they are, the more fluid they lose).

In a dehydrated state, exercises are harder to perform, stamina drops, heart rate increases and a young dancer may experience cramps, headaches and nausea. A good sign of hydration is the urine test: dark urine means they are dehydrated. Urine should be pale in colour.

Aim to be well hydrated before a class or performance, and encourage the young dancer to drink 6–8 cups (1–1.5 litres) of fluid each day – see Tables 7.3 and 7.4. Divide drinks into manageable quantities.

Table 7.3. Fluid requirements during exercise

30 minutes before exercise	During exercise	After exercise
150–200ml (1 glass)	100ml (½ glass) every 30 minutes	As much as is comfortable

Table 7.4. Choosing the best drink

Exercise less than 90 minutes	Exercise more than 90 minutes	To drink throughout the day
Water OR Fruit juice diluted 2 parts water to 1 part juice	Fruit juice diluted 1–2 parts water to 1 part juice	Where possible. If the young dancer finds it difficult to drink enough water, offer a flavoured drink (fruit juice diluted one or two parts water to one part fruit juice). Sugar-free squash or ordinary diluted squash is less expensive, but be aware that many brands contain additives, artificial sweeteners, colours and flavourings. Organic squashes are better options.

A healthy way to weight loss

Young dancers who are a healthy weight should not be encouraged to lose weight. If they are unhappy about their current size, the underlying problem could be related to low self-esteem, or perhaps they naturally have a larger frame and would not be suited to certain styles of dance, particularly ballet. This most certainly doesn't mean that all dance styles cannot be enjoyed as a recreation. Exercise appreciably improves posture, muscle tone and metabolic rate, and encourages creativity, artistry and fun!

If a young dancer's health or performance would benefit from reducing their fat percentage, follow the advice below, or alternatively seek the advice of a registered dietitian or nutritionist. A combination of exercise and healthy eating is all that is needed for healthy weight loss, and with professional guidance a young dancer should lose no more than 1–2kg per month (depending on age and weight). Leave at least 3 to 4 weeks between achieving the desired weight loss and an audition or rehearsal, as the slight restriction in calories could hinder the dancer's energy levels and skill. By following a healthy eating plan, the young dancer will not forfeit their health and development, and will be encouraged to follow a healthy lifestyle and attitude in the long term.

Dos and dont's for healthy weight loss

- Do tell the young dancer that you realise it is sometimes difficult to make healthy food choices.
- Don't tell them that they are lazy, greedy or fat, or need to lose weight.
- Don't make them feel ashamed of their eating habits.
- Do praise them generously when they make healthy choices.
- Do make them feel confident – a young dancer is much more likely to choose healthy foods when they feel positive about themselves. Emphasise their strengths and accomplishments.
- Don't say you are putting them on a diet. Just encourage them to eat healthily.
- Don't use food as a reward. Allow treats on a certain day of the week and after a meal.
- Do lead by example. Young dancers learn from their parents and elders, and eating the same food as them makes them realise that it is all about healthy eating in general, and that they do not need to follow a 'special' diet to keep them trim.
- Do provide healthy snacks instead of biscuits, cakes, chocolates, sweets and crisps. Keep stores topped up so that they are easily accessible and quick to prepare.
- Don't refuse any foods, but explain that they should be eaten only occasionally.
- Do encourage them to exercise outside of the dance class if they are particularly inactive the rest of the time.
  - 6–10-year-olds are encouraged to participate in 60 minutes of moderate-intensity exercise per day.
  - 11–15-year-olds are encouraged to participate in 30–60 minutes of moderate to vigorous activity per day PLUS 3 sessions per week of 20 minutes' continuous activity.
- Unless stated, exercise does not have to be done in one session. Recommendations include everyday activities such as walking, ball games, PE etc.

Healthy & handy eating tips

- Include five portions of fruit and vegetables a day.
- Choose low-fat dairy products. All the benefits of dairy foods are maintained, but with much less animal fat.
- Choose healthy snacks as listed.
- Follow the 'third of a plate' rule, whereby vegetables or salad should take up around a third of a plate. This will help to keep the dancer's diet balanced and will satisfy hunger.
- Include fruit for dessert, whether fresh, stewed or baked.
- Make healthier options (such as home-made burgers or thick chips) as an alternative to the unhealthy ones.
- For treats, choose fun-size chocolate bars instead of regular size.
- Include soup made with lots of vegetables, beans and lentils, as they are nutritious and filling.
- Choose wholemeal cereals and grains (wholegrain bread, bran cereals, porridge, whole-wheat pasta), because they satisfy hunger better than white versions. Swap over gradually, however, to avoid stomach upset and discomfort.

Restaurant meals and fast foods

The following fast foods are very tempting, but alas high in calories and saturated fat. Try to find healthy alternatives, and save the foods listed below for the occasional treat.

- Greasy burgers and chips
- Fried chicken or chicken nuggets
- Battered fish and chips
- Pasta/rice in creamy or oily sauces
- Pizzas topped with lots of cheese and fatty red meat
- Hot dogs.

Slow weight gain/growth

A good proportion of young dancers struggle to keep a healthy weight, because they burn a lot of energy during exercise. Here are a few tips on helping them to keep up healthily with growth and activity demands.

- Encourage slightly bigger portions at mealtimes.
- Encourage the young dancer to eat more frequent meals (particularly if they find it difficult to eat larger main meals).
- Include snacks that have a high concentration of energy (see the high-energy snacks listed below).
- Encourage manageable quantities of nutritious drinks such as milk, home-made milkshakes, yoghurt drinks or fruit smoothies.
- Sprinkle a little grated cheese on potatoes, rice and pasta dishes.
- Avoid filling up on biscuits, cakes and other puddings. They will provide calories, but these have little nutritional value (the foods are low in vitamins and minerals) and are high in unhealthy saturated/hydrogenated fats.
- Include milk-based or yoghurt-based puddings (rice pudding, fruit crumble with custard, banana or stewed apple and custard, bread pudding, mini egg custards).

High-energy snacks

- Nuts (peanuts, cashews, brazils, pistachios etc.)
- Dried fruit (raisins, sultanas, dates etc.)
- Scones, muffins, fruit buns, malt loaf
- Mini-bagels, mini-pancakes, rolls
- Healthy breakfast or cereal bars (avoid those covered in chocolate or frosted sugar)
- Wholemeal sandwiches and oatcakes with cheese or peanut butter
- Cheese on toast.

Summary

- A growing and developing body needs good nutrition; feeding the body is equally as important as training the body.
- Young dancers have higher energy needs than the mature dancer, as their bodies are growing and they 'waste' energy during dance because of inexperience.
- Dancers can meet their protein needs by including two to four portions of protein-rich food each day. This includes lean meat, fish, poultry, eggs, beans, nuts etc. Their requirements are around 1.1–1.2g per kg of bodyweight.

- Carbohydrate provides around 50 per cent of the dancer's diet, and is used to fuel dance and 'save' protein. To ensure a balanced diet, base a meal or snack around a carbohydrate, then decide on the protein.
- Young dancers should include small amounts of healthy fats (olive oil, oily fish, nuts and seeds) and limit saturated fats (fats predominantly of animal origin). Refer to Chapter 4 for more information on the importance of fat and how to get the right amount.
- Foods eaten before an event should be easily digested and familiar. Avoid trying new foods before an important event.
- Choose snacks high in carbohydrate to provide energy to sustain young dancers throughout an event. Do avoid high sugar snacks and drinks, however, as they can lead to fluctuations in blood sugars and energy levels.
- Young dancers are vulnerable to dehydration. Encourage 6–8 cups of fluid each day, and divide drinks into manageable amounts. Ensure dancers are well hydrated before exercise, but also that they have enough time to visit the bathroom beforehand.
- Dancers who are of a healthy weight should not be encouraged to lose weight. If the young dancer would benefit from weight loss, a combination of a healthy diet and exercise will help achieve this. They should lose no more than 1–2kg per month (depending on age and weight).
- By following a healthy eating plan, the young dancer will not forfeit their health, development and performance.

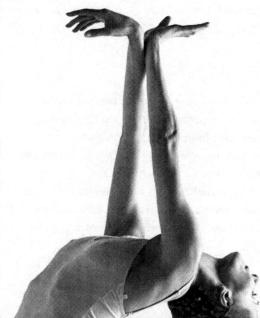

Rebecca Sewell: Dancer with Balletomane Theatre
Photograph © Phil Conrad

Chapter 8
The Mirror and the Dancer –
Body Sculpting and Weight Loss

The practice mirror is to be used for the correction of faults, not for a love affair, and the figure you watch should not become your dearest friend.

Agnes de Mille

Can a dancer really stay extremely slim, yet maintain a healthy diet and ultimately a healthy body? These questions have hovered precariously over the delicate line between a healthy body and a too-slender physique.

Undeniably, pressure to acquire a certain body shape has existed in all forms of dance, particularly as fashion has leant towards an extremely low percentage of body fat. Dance styles are known to differ in the amount of pressure placed on a certain body shape; ballet dancers in particular experience tremendous pressure to maintain a very low body-fat percentage. As competitive standards get higher, so does the necessity to strive for the leaner, more fashionable figure. And so significant is the shape and size of the body, that dancers may reduce their calorie intake and compromise their health for the desired figure. Dancers are more readily encouraged to diet than to participate in exercises specifically designed to reshape and sculpt the body.

Dancers are extremely vulnerable creatures. Their body and their art are intricately related, distinguishing them from artists, musicians and writers, who are able to distance themselves from their work and talents by putting down their paintbrushes, instruments and pens. Dancers use only their bodies. When dancers are told they are of the wrong shape, are too big or too fat or have bad feet, it is very difficult to take this as a criticism of their art rather than of themselves.

Addressing the predicament that faces dancers who forfeit a healthy diet in the pursuit of a lean body, numerous studies have confirmed that, although dancers need more calories than non-active people, they maintain their weight even when their calorie intake is below requirements. These findings strongly suggest that the dancer's body has adapted to a low calorie intake in an attempt to conserve energy whilst coping with the demands of intense exercise. Consequently, the dancer's metabolic rate is lowered, and weight remains fixed. It is therefore extremely important that dancers and supporters of dance recognise that an adequate diet that encourages a more efficient metabolic rate can help dancers achieve a lean physique far more successfully than one that forces the body to become sluggish and conserving. A metabolic rate that has been lowered through dietary restrictions can most definitely be restored – but by a process that must be gradually introduced into the dancer's diet over a period of time to allow the metabolic rate to increase gradually.

Dancers of course differ from one another, but it is very possible to maintain a lean physique and be healthy through a combination of good nutrition and exercise that shapes and moulds the contours of the dancer's body.

How much body fat should we have?

A certain amount of body fat is vital. First and foremost, fat is a constituent of cells, brain tissue, nerves and bone marrow, and also protects and cushions vital organs (heart, liver and kidneys). In total this accounts for about 3 per cent of your body weight, and is known as *essential fat*.

Women have an extra 'essential fat' requirement that accounts for an additional 5–9 per cent. This fat is stored in the breasts and around the hips, and is necessary for the production of oestrogen, which ensures a normal hormone balance and menstruation. The menstrual cycle can represent an external voice for internal circumstances. If the body is in chemical balance, then the dancer will experience regular menstrual periods. If the body is stressed, or lacking in some factor, then menstruation may stop: the body is not healthy enough to reproduce. If nutritional intake, body weight or exercise is putting the dancer's body under stress, this will most likely be demonstrated in menstrual regulation. A small amount of essential fat is also necessary for the normal hormone production in men.

Another type of body fat is known as *storage fat* and lies under the skin and around the organs. This fat is a source of energy, and is used nearly all the time for all activities (aerobic exercise, sleeping, standing, sitting, walking). The body tends to use fat from all the sites where it is stored, although individuals do vary because of differences in genetic makeup and the type of exercise they undertake.

For exercising individuals, physiologists recommend a minimum body fat level of 5 per cent for men and 12–14 per cent for women to cover the basic functions required for a healthy body (slim non-dancers are likely to have a body fat level of around 9–20 per cent for men and 21–31 per cent for women). On average, body fat percentages in female dancers lie between 11 and 21 per cent. Exercising individuals can fall below the percentages calculated for non-active individuals because they have a greater percentage of muscle, thus altering the ratio of body fat to lean body mass. Female dancers can still experience regular menstrual periods if their diet is balanced and sufficient; but note that the values above are absolute minima, and the optimal body fat percentage is closer to 8–12 per cent for men and 16–20 per cent for women. Additionally, every dancer is an individual, so what may be an appropriate level of body fat for one dancer may prove too low for another. Dancers who try to maintain a very low body fat level, or one that is unnatural for their own individual body, will encounter problems in both health and performance.

Note
Dancers can experience the loss of menstruation (amenorrhoea) for a combination of factors, including low body weight, low body fat, exercise intensity, anxiety, poor diet, low calorie intake and genetic makeup. It is vitally important for dancers and supporters of dance to assess all areas of the dancer's lifestyle in order to correctly determine the true cause of amenorrhoea (a dancer may regain her periods just by following a healthier diet rather than needing to gain bodyweight or body fat). Once the true cause is established, dancers, teachers and parents can then help make lifestyle changes to correct the health issue.

What is a BMI?

BMI stands for Body Mass Index, and represents an additional method of analysing a dancer's health. BMI determines what weight a dancer should be for their given height:

$$BMI = \frac{Weight\ (Kg)}{[Height\ (m)]^2}$$

The value determines whether the dancer is underweight, normal weight or overweight, as defined by the World Health Organisation – see Table 8.1.

Table 8.1. BMI classification

Less than 18.4	Underweight
18.5–24.9	Normal weight
25–29.9	Overweight
30–40	Moderately obese
40+	Severely obese

How to work out your BMI

Step 1: Work out your weight in kg (refer to Chapter 1 for how to convert stones and pounds to kilograms).

Step 2: Work out your height in metres (1 foot = 0.3048 metres, 1 inch = 0.0254 metres).

Example.
Suppose a dancer has a weight of 54kg and a height of 5ft 6 inches. Converting that to metres, 5ft × 0.3048 PLUS 6 inches × 0.0254 = 1.68 metres.

$$BMI = \frac{54kg}{1.68m^2} = 19.1 kg/m^2$$

I have calculated my BMI, but don't think it puts me in the right category.

The BMI chart is a guideline designed for health professionals to assess the general public's health and risk of disease. Although BMI is a useful tool for dancers, teachers and parents, it is just one method, and advice given must not be based solely on the BMI. This is not to say that BMI charts are not useful indicators, but many dancers and other active individuals have body compositions that are dissimilar to those of the general public, and the BMI charts do not take this into account. They must be used in conjunction with other risk factors (body fat percentage, exercise intensity, stress, dietary habits) in the prevention of injury, osteoporosis and amenorrhoea. In individuals who undertake regular exercise, measuring body fat may provide a more accurate determination of health and body shape.

What is 'body composition'?

'Body composition' is a phrase used to describe what the human body is composed of. We know that it contains bone, muscle, fat, ligaments and so on, but that does not give us an idea of how much there is of each component. So, as a way to illustrate the shape of a dancer, we can describe their 'body composition'.

When BMI doesn't tell you all: A tale of two dancers

Why do these two dancers look different? They have the same weight and height.

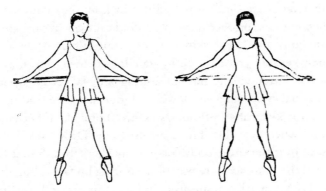

Figure 8. Dancer 1: weight 52kg, body fat 22%   Figure 9. Dancer 2: weight 52kg, body fat 17%

They look different because dancer 1 has more fat but less muscle compared with dancer 2, and therefore her body composition is different. This gives them different body shapes even though their body weights are the same. This is an example of where body weight doesn't always give us an accurate impression of a dancer's shape, physique and health.

And another thing......

Even though these two dancers weigh the same, dancer 1 needs slightly fewer calories than dancer 2 does, as she has less muscle. Muscle needs more energy to maintain itself than fat does.

Final question: Does a balanced diet encourage greater lean muscle and less body fat? Answer: Most definitely yes!

Measuring and reducing body fat

There are several different techniques for determining body fat percentage: examples include using skinfold callipers, bioelectrical impedance analysis and dual energy x-ray absorptiometry (DEXA).

Skinfold callipers measure the layer of fat underneath the skin by pinching selected parts of the body (usually triceps, biceps, hip bone, lower back, abdomen, thigh and below the shoulder blade). Accuracy depends on the person performing the skinfold test, and dancers tend to have a different fat distribution from that of non-dancers. This method is accurate to within 3–4 per cent body fat.

Bioelectrical impedance analysis is used in most body fat monitors and scales. It works by sending a very mild electrical current through the body, using the fact that fat, water and muscle differ in how they conduct electricity. This method has the same accuracy as skinfold callipers (results are affected by changes in body fluid and skin temperature). When using this form of measurement, ensure you are well hydrated, as dehydration may give you a higher body fat measurement. Also, measuring body fat percentage immediately after a menstrual cycle will give a lower and more accurate reading.

Dual energy x-ray absorptiometry (DEXA) provides information on total body fat and where it is distributed on the body. DEXA involves two types of X-ray scan over the entire body. Taking anywhere from 5 to 20 minutes to perform, it is the most accurate way of measuring body fat, but also the most expensive. DEXA machines are usually found in research institutions and hospitals.

Reducing the percentage of body fat

Body fat is stored within fat cells, the size of which is determined by how much fat we have. The distribution and quantity of fat cells around the body is largely dictated by our gender and genetic makeup (for example, you are likely to have a body shape similar to your mother's or father's). There is very little you can do to affect the way the body distributes fat, or even how many fat cells you have; but you can greatly affect how much fat is stored in them.

In order to lose weight, we basically need to take in fewer calories than our body requires. Our own fat stores will then be used to keep us going.

The body first recognises a modest reduction in calories, and will start using stored fat as a result. If your diet becomes too restrictive and you cut your calories too radically, your body will be encouraged to lower its metabolic rate in an attempt to reserve energy. A very low-calorie diet certainly doesn't mean you lose weight more quickly. Muscle breakdown occurs, thus further reducing your metabolic rate (less muscle means that you need fewer calories to maintain your weight).

To ensure that your weight loss is due to losing body fat and not lean muscle, aim to lose no more than 0.5–1lb per week. To do this, you will need to reduce your daily calorie intake by about 15–20 per cent. In most cases, this is equivalent to around 300–400kcal each day. For example, if you require 2000kcal per day to maintain your current weight, that means you need to reduce your intake by about 300-400kcal, making your new calorie requirement 1600–1700kcal per day.

Weight loss plan
- Reduce calorie intake by 15–20 per cent to achieve steady and gradual weight loss.
- Maintain, or even gain, lean muscle mass.
- Gradually reduce your body fat percentage.
- Avoid reducing your resting metabolic rate (see Chapter 1).
- Ensure your diet is balanced and your performance does not suffer.

Where to start?!

Even though you need to reduce your total calorie intake, your diet must still be balanced and include all the nutrients necessary for your performance not to suffer (don't forget, exercise will also help you to achieve a trim physique).

Carbohydrate

Now that you have moderately reduced your daily intake, carbohydrate should contribute around 50 per cent of your total calories: to fuel exercise, to encourage the body to burn fat when dancing, and to prevent lean muscle loss. If you reduce your carbohydrate intake too much, you run the risk of sacrificing energy levels, technique and skill, and you are likely to feel tired and drained ... and lacking lustre! Still aim to base meals and snacks on a good source of carbohydrate – just take care that it is not served with anything high in fat. To ensure you are getting the right balance, carbohydrate should take up a third of your plate, or a third of the meal.

Protein

When you eat fewer calories than your body needs to maintain its weight, it will automatically start using its own stores of energy to keep going. Stored body fat is obviously the preferred choice, but there is always the opportunity for your body to use protein from muscle instead. To prevent this from happening, dancers reducing their weight need slightly more protein than those maintaining their weight. This is just to ensure that weight loss is down to a reduction in body fat and not in muscle. In other words, you should maintain or slightly increase your protein intake (see Table 8.2), and slightly reduce your carbohydrate intake. Of your total intake, carbohydrate then contributes 50 per cent (rather than up to 60 per cent) and protein around 25 per cent (15–20 per cent normally being recommended for weight maintenance).

Table 8.2. Protein requirements per day

Weight maintenance	1.2–1.6g per kg bodyweight / day
Weight loss	1.6–2.0g per kg bodyweight / day

Example
A dancer weighing 60kg on a weight loss programme.
Protein requirements: 60kg × 1.6g/kg = 96g
60kg × 2.0g/kg = 120g
So the dancer should eat 96–120g protein each day.

Tip
Aim to include protein in two meals each day – it should take up a third of the plate, or a third of a meal. You can also choose snacks that offer a good portion of protein, such as low-fat dairy products or small quantities of chicken with crispbread.

Tip
Always choose low-fat options of protein – they provide at least as much protein as higher-fat protein sources do.

Fat

This is the main area that you want to be strict with. Fat has 9 kcal per gram, over twice the number of calories as the same weight of carbohydrate or protein. So cutting it down is the most efficient way of reducing your calorie intake without having to restrict carbohydrate too much or sacrifice protein – both of which are very important for performance, body composition, achieving the desired body shape and metabolism.

Do still include small amounts of healthy fats (oily fish, nuts and seeds, olive oil), as they are vitally important for injury avoidance, flexible joints and keeping colds and flu at bay.

Unhealthy fats are the ones to look out for; they do not contribute to greater energy levels nor to lean, toned muscles; and when you are trying to reduce your body fat, leave these fats on the supermarket shelves. The odd treat, of course, is allowed!

Fluid

Here is yet another reason why fluid is vital for the dancer. Not only does water improve performance and energy levels (see Chapter 6), but in terms of reducing body fat it is absolutely necessary for a good metabolism. It keeps muscles and skin toned, and helps to reduce water retention by stimulating your kidneys to flush out toxins that can accumulate and lead to excess fluid being carried around the body.

Water retention can be caused by:

- regularly eating too much salt or sugar
- not eating enough fresh fruit and vegetables
- high levels of wastes or toxins in your body
- taking certain commonly prescribed medications
- long-term use of very low-calorie diets, which tend to be low in protein and other important nutrients
- food intolerances.

Drink water where possible, but other options such as fruit and herbal teas, sugar-free squashes and diet drinks are also a good way of taking in fluid.

The Top Ten Tips (and one more)

1. **Aim to lose 0.5kg (1lb) a week – and no more.**
   This may not sound much, but if you want to maintain your metabolic rate, lose fat and maintain lean muscle mass, this is most definitely the right way. Faster weight loss could result in lean muscle loss, and it would become increasingly hard not only to continue losing fat, but also to keep the weight off.

   Note that you may lose as much as 2kg in the first week or so, because of a small loss in glycogen and fluid.

2. **Aim for the right type of weight loss for the right reason.**
   Before starting a weight loss programme, set a goal that is manageable and attainable. For instance, you may want to lose 5kg (11lb) in body fat, and have set a clear time frame of around 10–11 weeks.

   Also think about why you are trying to lose weight: is it to be a more suitable weight for your frame? Is it to fall within the body fat threshold for a dancer?

3. **Monitor your body shape and body composition.**
   You don't necessarily have to jump on the scales to notice a difference; how your clothes fit is a very good indicator of how your body shape is changing, and simple measurements taken around the waist, hip and thigh areas (the main areas where fat is stored) will also give you an accurate idea of whether you are losing body fat. Weigh yourself no more than once a week, and don't be disheartened if you haven't lost any weight in some weeks: it may just be that you have gained a little muscle and may actually look leaner!

4. **Don't go below your resting metabolic rate (RMR).**
   The body is very good at adapting; so if you eat less than you need, your body will just slow down, fall into a 'survival' mode and use fewer calories. This is not particularly helpful when you are (a) trying to lose weight, (b) wanting to perform at your best, and (c) wanting to achieve your ideal physique. Sticking to a 15–20 per cent reduction in total calories will prove the most successful way. Chapter 1 explained how to estimate your personal RMR.

5. **Write it down!**
   Sometimes it helps to write down (maybe one day a week) what you have eaten that day, to check that it is balanced, and that you are eating enough protein and not too much unhealthy fat. This exercise

does not need to be done every day, just on the odd occasion to keep you on the right track!

6. **Skim away unhealthy fats.**

    Choosing low-fat dairy products and lean protein will help to keep unhealthy fats at an all-time low whilst ensuring you are getting all the benefits in terms of health, dance and weight loss. Limiting the amount of pastries, cakes, biscuits and processed savoury foods will also be of enormous benefit in terms of reducing body fat. Replace these tempting foods with low-fat but equally tasty alternatives.

7. **Make a little room for healthy fats.**

    Small amounts of healthy fats are important for healthy skin, hair, flexible joints, keeping colds at bay, and that old brain matter. Including oily fish once or twice a week, and using a tablespoon of olive oil as a dressing (vegetable oil when cooking) should do the trick.

8. **More is less – add volume!**

    Including lots of salad and vegetables of all kinds is a wondrous way of keeping trim, ensuring you are getting plenty of rich nutrients, and pleasing your appetite. Add salads and vegetables with meals, and snack on fruit between meals and classes.

9. **Get enough protein.**

    Protein often gets the raw end of the deal when it comes to reducing calorie intake; and you actually need a little more protein than if you were maintaining your weight. Your body is always tempted to use protein from its own stores (muscle), so, to ensure it's fat you're losing and not muscle, include 2–4 portions of lean protein each day (equivalent to a third of your plate or meal). Protein also helps to control appetite, and a meal containing protein makes you feel more satisfied.

10. **Take little steps.**

    Small regular meals and snacks will help to control your appetite and prevent food cravings, so try to eat four to six times a day at regular intervals. You might do this with a combination of three meals (breakfast, lunch and evening meal) and a few small snacks in between. Regular eating also has a positive effect on the metabolic rate, keeps energy levels up, and is satisfying!

And lastly:

11. The little gems ...

When you feel a little hungry, and need a snack to keep you going till the next meal, the following little nibbles are healthy, low in fat, and, most importantly, tasty.

Small snacks
- Wholemeal English muffins, fruit buns and plain scones with a little low-fat spread, yeast extract or light cream cheese
- Oat/Scotch/home-made pancakes
- Crispbread, oatcakes and rice cakes with a healthy topping (such as light cream cheese, low-fat hummus, cottage cheese, or chicken or ham slices)
- Fruit
- Carrot, cucumber and celery sticks with a healthy dip
- Low-fat yoghurts and low-fat fromage frais
- Smoothies with crushed fruit and low-fat yoghurt.

Moderate-sized snacks
- Baked beans on toast (add yeast extract or Tabasco sauce for flavour, and avoid butter and cheese)
- A handful of dried fruit and nuts
- Wholemeal sandwich, roll, pitta bread, bagel or toast with a healthy filling.

Summary

- Through a combination of exercise and a balanced diet, dancers do not have to sacrifice their health in order to achieve their ideal body shape.
- A minimum of 5–12 per cent body fat is healthy in male dancers, and 12–20 per cent in female dancers. This is significantly lower than for a slim non-dancer.
- BMI charts are a convenient way of estimating a healthy weight, but should not be used on their own to determine a dancer's health and well-being.
- Body fat percentage can be measured using skin callipers, bioelectrical impedance analysis and DEXA.

- Never consume less than your RMR (resting metabolic rate) requirements, as doing so will have a negative effect on metabolism, health and performance.
- In a balanced diet, 50 per cent should come from carbohydrates, 25 per cent from protein and 25 per cent from fat. Dancers aiming to reduce body fat have slightly higher protein requirements and slightly lower carbohydrate requirements.
- Aim to include four to six meals per day (three meals and one to three snacks) to maintain a healthy metabolic rate and avoid fluctuating blood sugars.
- Follow the 'third of a plate' rule (or 'third of a meal' rule!) – a third carbohydrate, a third protein and a third salad/vegetables.

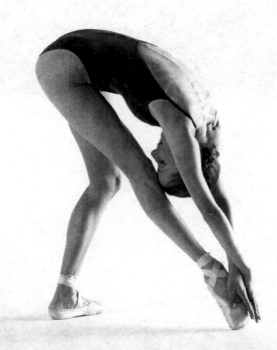

Dancer: Rebecca Sewell
Photograph © Phil Conrad

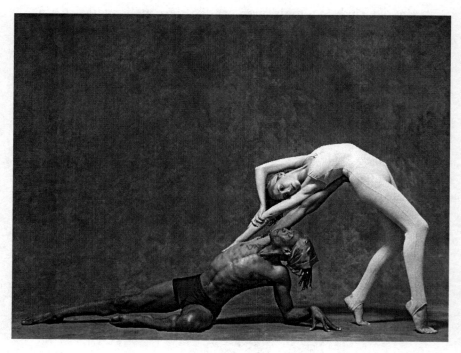

Photograph © Eric Richmond

Chapter 9
Fad Diets

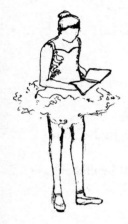

The mirror is not you. The mirror is you looking at yourself.

George Balanchine

The definition of a fad diet is rather subjective. The term 'fad' is often used to describe diets that are extreme, claim miracle weight loss and go against advice from health professionals. However, a fad diet can quite simply be a weight loss plan that becomes very popular (quickly) and then may fail (quickly) to provide long-term, healthy weight loss.

Recognising a fad diet

Fad diets often use the words 'easy', 'effortless', 'guaranteed', 'miraculous', 'breakthrough', 'mysterious', 'exotic', 'exclusive' or 'secret', or phrases such as 'New discovery', 'Eat all you want and still lose weight!', 'Melt away the fat whilst you sleep' or 'Lose 30lb in 30 days!'.

So what is it that are you mostly lose when following radical diets or those that 'contradict health professional advice'? The answer is water, glycogen stores and lean muscle mass.

Phrases from nutritionists characterising a fad diet

- Eliminates one or more of the five food groups (starch, protein, fat, dairy, fruit and vegetables)
- Encourages an imbalanced diet
- Promises a 'quick fix' or rapid weight loss (more than 2lb per week)
- Comments that the diet may appear 'too good to be true'
- Bases recommendations on the product being sold
- Uses celebrities to endorse the diet
- Lists 'good' foods and 'bad' foods
- Are accompanied by dramatic statements likely to be refuted by reputable, well-known scientific organisations
- Offers claims of success based on testimonies from other dieters and their own scientific explanations rather than using studies from recognised scientific organisations
- Doesn't encourage or promote exercise as part of a healthy lifestyle.

Common problems with fad diets

Imbalanced diets may recommend that carbohydrate, protein and fat be eaten in quantities that contradict advice from nutritionists and dietitians. Weight loss may be experienced initially; but because the diet does not provide the right quantities of each nutrient, the body will adjust, producing a negative effect on metabolism, health and, for the dancer, performance. Do copious amounts of fat-laden cheese and fatty meat sound healthy to you?

A rapid weight loss diet based on an exotic-sounding herb supplement cannot aid weight loss when the diet is high in fat and sugar. Natural and safe herbs and supplements may subtly promote a healthier metabolic rate, but dramatic claims of rapid weight loss can be dangerous and untrue. And short-term.

A low-calorie diet encourages the body to lower the metabolic rate in order to conserve energy, especially if calorie intake falls below the resting metabolic rate (see Chapter 1). Ultimately, this just makes it harder to lose weight or keep weight off. Our bodies are very good at adapting to our environment: the less you eat; the less you need. (Thankfully, a reduced metabolic rate can be successfully reversed when foods are introduced gradually and exercise is incorporated.)

A restrictive diet that eliminates or avoids certain food groups will not only be difficult to follow in the long term, but also encourage nutritional deficiencies that would affect health, performance and metabolism. Weight is often regained once the diet is no longer followed, and in many cases subjects weigh more than when they started the diet, as their metabolism has been affected.

A miracle diet not backed by scientific studies may nevertheless seem logical in some cases, but claims are often based on basic knowledge that has been altered slightly to create a statement that is no longer accurate. You cannot put 2 and 2 together to make 5.5.

Yo-yo dieting is a term used to describe dieting practices whereby a person may undertake severe food restriction and fasting, followed by overeating. Each time the person stops dieting, weight returns, and often the dieter weighs more than ever before. When you fast or severely restrict your intake for long periods of time, the body 'reserves' energy. When you overeat, the body is much more likely to store those calories as body fat, as it thinks it may experience another episode of fasting (your body has a good memory!). Body weight fluctuates, and metabolism is affected.

> **A fad fact**
> Only 5 per cent of dieters keep weight off in the long term.

Different ways of losing weight

In a **healthy balanced diet**, focus is placed on reducing weight whilst promoting long-term lifestyle changes that encourage long-term successful results, healthily. There is no need to change the types of food eaten once the person's ideal weight is reached.

In a **fad diet**, focus is placed on quick, flash-style weight loss for short-term and (semi-) successful results – and, most often, unhealthily. The diet cannot be sustained on a long-term basis.

Ironically, it is often the fad diet that can be labelled 'long and boring'. It can become tedious and repetitive owing to its restriction or elimination of certain foods.

If a diet is restrictive, avoids certain food groups, is imbalanced, has a very low calorie intake or is based on a miracle herb, it is very unlikely to work in the long term. Restrictive diets cannot be followed over a long period, so dieters often regain weight because they do not know what they should be eating once the diet is stopped. Additionally, rapid weight loss and excessive calorie restriction result in muscle loss and a slower metabolism, making it harder to keep the weight off. Moreover, the body has by then adopted a 'survival' mechanism, and needs fewer calories to carry out everyday functions. It is also very likely that the dieter has become deficient in many different vitamins and minerals, and will not be performing at their best. They may feel energised and healthy at the beginning of the diet, but unfortunately this is not long-lasting, and the consequences of a poor diet will be just around the corner!

Fortunately, the effects of a restrictive diet can be reversed in most cases, and a gradual introduction of a varied diet, combined with exercise, will correct nutritional deficiencies and encourage the metabolic rate to function effectively.

Using laxatives is another, rather drastic, method of weight loss; but they only manage to dehydrate the body and make food rush through the large intestine more quickly. Laxatives do not prevent calories being absorbed. The large colon (where laxatives operate) does not absorb major nutrients, but only water, salt, B vitamins and soluble fibre – food for 'friendly bacteria'. Laxatives therefore dehydrate. Performance suffers and many metabolic activities struggle to cope, and become sluggish.

The most popular diets

The Zone Diet

This idea of a relaxed metabolic and mental 'zone' was created by Barry Sears.
Principle: 40% carbohydrate, 30% protein, 30% fat
Claims to:

- promote weight loss
- increase mental focus
- increase physical performance.

What the experts point out:

- Very strict quantities of food portioned into blocks at particular times of day.
- Unhealthy attitude to foods by categorising foods as good or bad rather than 'eat plenty of' or 'just small amounts of'.
- Total calories averaged at 1300kcal – some menus are as low as 850kcal per day, making it a very low-calorie diet in disguise. Many menus fall

below the resting metabolic rate (see Chapter 1), thus reducing the metabolic rate and making it hard to keep the weight off.
- Relies on unproven claims that have not been published in scientific journals.

Short-term weight loss? Yes
Long-term weight loss? No
Long and tedious? Yes!

The Atkins Diet

Created by Dr Robert Atkins as a rebellion against the 1980s diet trend of all things carbohydrate!

Principle: Without carbohydrate in the diet, the body is forced to use fat for energy – therefore the diet is almost all protein and fat (of any sort). This forces the body into ketosis (see below), which is how you lose weight.

Claims to:

- promote rapid weight loss
- increase energy levels
- reduce appetite.

What the experts point out:

- Very limited food choice (difficult to follow in the long term).
- No published scientific studies and trials to support the claims behind the diet.
- Nutritionally imbalanced and excessively high in protein, fat and processed foods.
- Very low in calcium, vitamin C, folic acid and several other vitamins and minerals.
- Dehydration very possible if large quantities of water are not drunk.
- Weight loss is accredited to dehydration, loss of glycogen stores, lean muscle and some body fat. If 60 per cent of our body is water, that's quite a big weight loss (and weight gain afterwards)!
- Without carbohydrate, fat cannot be completely broken down. Instead it forms by-products called ketones, which can cause considerable damage to vital organs when present in large quantities.

In order to prevent these substances from building up in the blood with nowhere to go, the body is forced to excrete them through urine, sweat and breath, resulting in bad breath, dizziness, migraines, nausea and weakness.

Short-term weight loss? Yes
Long-term weight loss? No
Long and tedious? Of course!

The Grapefruit Diet

Created in 1930s Hollywood, and one of the oldest and most discussed Hollywood fad diets.

Principle: Involves large quantities of grapefruit and small amounts of black coffee, the odd piece of dry toast, egg and, when generous, fish or meat in the evening. Calorie intake is restricted to about 800kcal per day. It is based on the idea that grapefruit has 'fat-burning enzymes'.

Claims to:

• promote rapid weight loss.

What the experts point out:

• Very narrow range of foods.
• Imbalanced diet leading to many nutrient deficiencies.
• Grapefruit has no 'fat burning powers'.
• No scientific basis to claim that grapefruit has these 'special' properties. It is a healthy food along with other fruits and vegetables.
• A very low-calorie diet, which results in a lowered metabolic rate.
• Does not promote healthy eating; therefore once the diet is abandoned, weight is often regained, and dieters often weigh more than when they started the diet.

Short-term weight loss? Yes
Long-term weight loss? No
Long and tedious? Most definitely!

The Cabbage Soup Diet: The 7-Day Diet

Principle: First introduced in the 1980s, this diet involves eating unlimited amounts of cabbage-based soup for 7 days. Limited other foods are allowed (Day 1 can also have fruit, Day 2 can have vegetables).
    Claims to:

- promote rapid weight loss.

What the experts point out:

- Very imbalanced diet leading to many nutrient deficiencies.
- One cannot lose 10lb of fat in 7 days. Weight loss is most likely due to loss of water, muscle and body fat.
- A very low-calorie diet, which lowers the metabolic rate.
- Does not promote healthy eating; so, once again, after 7 days, water lost during the diet is regained, and the dieter is likely to overeat on unhealthy foods, thus gaining more weight.

    Short-term weight loss? Yes
    Long-term weight loss? No
    Long and tedious? Goes without saying

The F-Plan Diet

Created by Audrey Eyton in 1982 – the first and most famous high-fibre diet.
    Principle: A high intake of dietary fibre fills you up and helps control appetite, thus preventing overeating. A typical diet is 1250kcal, and is low in fat, is high in complex carbohydrates, and has double the recommended amount of fibre each day (36g instead of 18g).
    Claims to:

- promote weight loss.

What the experts point out:

- People unused to high fibre may at first experience slight fluid retention.

- Straightforward diet that is fairly simple to prepare, with not too many rules.
- Some side effects such as bloating and flatulence, although they tend to pass.
- Must include plenty of water.
- Generally one of the healthiest diets around, and does encourage healthy eating principles.
- Tends to be low in essential fats such as omega oils (which are particularly important for the dancer).

Short-term weight loss? Yes
Long-term weight loss? Yes, but dancers must ensure that they are taking in enough calories to prevent muscle loss and fatigue.
Long and tedious? This diet is quite manageable if you can tolerate high-fibre foods without any unpleasant side effects!

The South Beach Diet

Created by Arthur Agatston.
   Principle: The South Beach Diet has three phases, and emphasises 'good' carbohydrates and 'good' fats. Phase I is followed for 2 weeks, phase II is followed until you have reached your target weight, and phase III is for weight maintenance and is therefore followed indefinitely.
   Claims to:

- promote weight loss
- promote a healthy-eating lifestyle.

What the experts point out:

- Phase I is a variation of the Atkins diet. Yet although it is high in protein and very low in carbohydrate, the diet is low in unhealthy fats (unlike the Atkins diet, which is high in fat).
- Phase II gradually introduces wholegrain foods, fruit and dairy products, encouraging a balanced diet.
- Phase III is based on a healthy balanced diet, and encourages a long-term healthy-eating lifestyle.
- Does not require calorie counting or limited servings.
- Several scientific studies have shown favourable results.

NOTE: Phase I could promote lean muscle loss, dehydration and fatigue in dancers owing to the very low intake of carbohydrate.

Short-term weight loss? Yes
Long-term weight loss? Yes
Long and tedious? No

WeightWatchers Diet

Principle: Based on a points system under which dieters are allowed a certain number of points per day. Foods are therefore categorised as 'good' or 'bad'.
  Claims to:

- promote weight loss
- be easy to follow
- allow you to eat the foods you like.

What the experts point out:

- Gradually reduces calories to 1000kcal per day, which is not sufficient to obtain all nutrients if the diet is followed for too long. Also, this falls below the resting metabolic rate, thus running the risk of reducing metabolism and making weight loss more difficult (see Chapter 1).
- Does not encourage a balanced diet, as you can eat whatever you choose as long as it adds up to the right number of points.
- Encourages dieters to think some foods are 'bad' and some are 'good'.

Short-term weight loss? Yes
Long-term weight loss? No – dieters often regain weight because their diet is still not balanced.
Long and tedious? Categorising food into 'points' can be very tedious, although some dieters have had positive results because they have designated points in such a way that their diet has become balanced and they have therefore been able to follow a varied diet.

So ...
  From the list above, it is clear that some fad diets are wildly extreme and very imaginative, while others are quite similar to what health professionals consider to be a balanced diet. Many other fad diets are available on the

internet, in books and in magazines: the Cambridge Diet, Slim Fast, ... the list is endless. However, just because a diet has a name doesn't always mean it is unhealthy. In the end, the best diet is a balanced diet – and your body will be more than happy to agree with you.

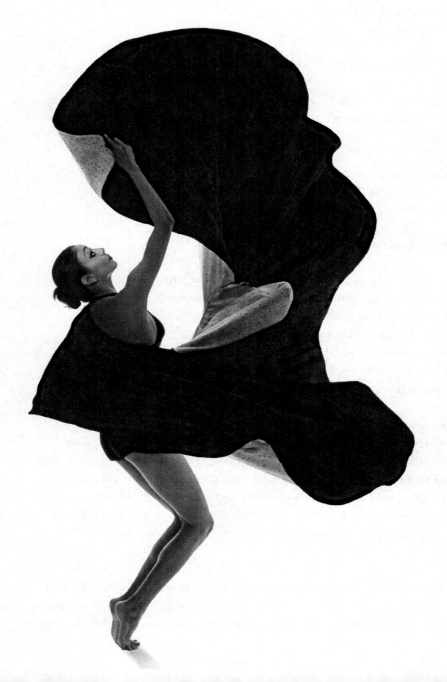

Photograph © Eric Richmond

Chapter 10
Irritable Bowel Syndrome, Food Intolerances and Sensitivities

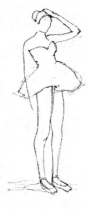

And those who were seen dancing were thought to be insane by those who could not hear the music.

Friedrich Wilhelm Nietzsche

Irritable Bowel Syndrome (IBS) is a condition that does not just affect the digestive system. There isn't, in fact, a single part of the body that escapes the symptoms of IBS. Also referred to as a 'functional' complaint, IBS presents as a disorder in the functioning of the digestive system, and not as an abnormality in its structure.

What causes IBS is still unclear, but developing the complaint is a very familiar way for a stressed body to react to a stressful lifestyle. A digestive system that harbours angst and tension will become bloated and painful and could lead to bouts of constipation and diarrhoea. The whole body will also suffer the consequences of a stressed digestive system: muscle aches, headaches, tiredness, backache, poor tolerance to pain, inability to concentrate and low morale. Your body may be stressed by the amount of exercise you are doing, by travel, through lack of sleep, or because of the things you eat.

Exacerbating factors for IBS

Stress can certainly make the symptoms of IBS worse, and can in some cases be the main reason why the digestive system constantly plays up. It is important therefore to try and reduce stressful situations, or discover ways in which to cope with a stressful event such as performance, audition and exam nerves.

If you know you are likely to get stressed around these events, choose low-risk foods that will help alleviate your symptoms.

IBS can be a mild annoyance, or something that notably affects your everyday activities. Some sufferers have to take several days, if not weeks, off work, but others experience very mild symptoms. So IBS can vary tremendously from one individual to another, and can be exacerbated by several different factors:

- Lifestyle: eating quickly, eating on the run, drinking fluids with meals, irregular meals, long periods of time without eating, dehydration
- Certain foods: spicy food, fatty food, fibrous foods, onions, mushrooms, cabbage, cauliflower, beans and pulses
- Certain fluids: fizzy drinks, caffeine, alcohol, sugary drinks, pure fruit juices
- Smoking
- Food intolerances: e.g. wheat, dairy, citrus fruits
- Overuse of antibiotics, antacids, laxatives and some medications.

When you are battling with the symptoms of IBS, you may need to limit or avoid certain foods or drinks. This doesn't necessarily mean that these particular foods are causing your symptoms, but they are aggravating them, and thus avoiding them will help reduce discomfort. When you are free of symptoms, you will most likely be able to include these foods again in your diet.

If you think you may have IBS, look through the possible triggers to determine which foods may be aggravating your digestive system, then make the necessary adjustments to your lifestyle and eating habits. Here are a few pointers:

Symptom: *Constipation*
  Cause: Possibly a sign of a low-fibre diet.
  Action:

- Try to include more wholegrain foods (wholemeal bread, wholegrain breakfast cereals) and increase your intake of fruit and vegetables.
- Introduce fibre gradually so that the body can become accustomed to it.
- Include a probiotic yoghurt drink or supplement to help balance the bacteria in the gut.
- Very importantly, drink plenty of fluids.

Symptom: *Diarrhoea*

Cause: Possibly aggravated by fibrous food, or too much of a particular food.

Action:

- Temporarily reduce the amount of fibre-rich foods (wholegrains, salads, fruits) and opt for low-fibre alternatives (white rice, white bread, peeled fruit, bananas, carrots, parsnips, swede).
- Limit the amount of fatty foods, and choose low-fat alternatives.
- Avoid spicy dishes.
- Limit alcohol, caffeine and fizzy drinks.
- Include a probiotic yoghurt drink or supplement to help recolonise bacteria in the gut.
- Include one or two portions of oily fish per week (salmon, sardines, mackerel, fish oil supplement) to help reduce inflammation.
- Certain foods containing pips, seeds and tough skins and stalks may cause problems and therefore may need to be avoided.
- Drink plenty of fluids.

Symptoms: *General IBS symptoms* such as bloating, pain, excessive wind, constipation and/or diarrhoea.

Cause: A number of possibilities, including lifestyle, eating habits, certain foods and food intolerances.

Action:

- Take time whilst eating, and avoid eating on the run.
- Eat regular meals or light snacks to avoid long periods of time without a meal.
- Include more or less high-fibre foods, depending on symptoms.
- Avoid high-risk foods and fluids such as fatty or spicy foods, alcohol, fizzy drinks and caffeine.
- Include a probiotic drink or supplement.
- Include one or two portions of oily fish each week.
- Drink plenty of fluids.

Herbal help and other medications

Some natural remedies can help combat the symptoms of IBS. Always follow the dosage instructions, as the powerful effects of plants and herbs can easily be underestimated!

Peppermint oil is a natural and effective way of managing symptoms

Aloe vera in liquid or tablet form is a natural and effective way of reducing inflammation and digestive discomfort. Make sure that the aloe vera supplement includes the leaf (to which the health benefits are accredited) rather than just the stalk.

Certain **medicines** help relax the muscles in the wall of the gut, and these are known as *antispasmodics*. Your doctor may advise an antispasmodic if you have spasm-type pains. There are several types of antispasmodic, each working in a slightly different way; so if you find that one type does not work for you, it is worth trying a different one. When you find a particular one that helps, take it 'as required' when pain symptoms flare up. Many people take an antispasmodic medicine for a week or so at a time to control pain when bouts of pain occur. Others take a dose before meals if pains tend to develop after eating.

Pains may ease with medication but may not go away completely. If you decide to take some antispasmodics, it is also important to look at your diet and lifestyle to see if you can establish the root cause.

IBS is painful but not serious. If you experience further, more serious symptoms such as unexplained fever, unexplained weight loss, abdominal pain, diarrhoea that disrupts night-time sleep, or rectal bleeding, seek medical attention.

Food intolerances and sensitivities

Food allergies occur when the immune system reacts to a certain food. Symptoms usually happen immediately after the offending food is eaten, and can range from serious reactions involving the throat and airways, to less serious effects such as digestive discomfort, skin irritation and headaches. Food allergies affect 2 per cent of the population, and sufferers must avoid all contact with the offending food, as minute quantities can initiate an allergic reaction.

Food intolerances, unlike food allergies, do not involve the immune system. Sufferers can often take in small amounts of the offending food, but larger quantities can lead to complaints such as digestive discomfort and skin reactions. Symptoms occur either several minutes after the food is eaten, or in the days following. Intolerances affect up to 40 per cent of the population, and can be self-inflicted (through eating large quantities of the same food) or genetic. The most common problem foods include wheat, dairy products and citrus fruits.

How can I tell if I have a food intolerance?

A simple and accurate way of diagnosing a food intolerance is to avoid the offending food for about two weeks. If symptoms improve, then it is likely that you have developed a food intolerance. If you see no improvement, then gradually reintroduce the food back into the diet, as there is no need to avoid it (unless it is unhealthy!).

NOTE: take out only one food group or item at a time (e.g. wheat, dairy etc). If you avoid more than one food, you will not know which one was causing the symptoms. Importantly, you need to substitute the troublesome food with an alternative, as your diet could become imbalanced and deficiencies are likely to occur.

A helping hand

The most effective way of managing a food intolerance or preventing one developing is to follow a varied, healthy diet. If you think you do not tolerate wheat very well, for example, you may be able to eat small amounts if you also include rice, potatoes, oats and corn-based foods. This way, you are not eating a lot of wheat each day (e.g. take a wheat-based breakfast, followed by bread for lunch and pasta for your evening meal).

Summary

- One in five people in the UK suffer from IBS.
- Typical symptoms include bloating, pain, excess wind, constipation, diarrhoea, headaches, muscles aches, back pain, tiredness, poor concentration and general lethargy.
- Sufferers of IBS may be symptom-free, followed by several days to weeks of discomfort.
- IBS may not necessarily be caused by, but can be made worse by, our lifestyles, certain foods, fluids, smoking, food intolerances and stress.
- The symptoms of IBS can be controlled through diet, medication or a combination of both.
- Symptoms vary greatly between individuals, and so it is often a process of trial and error to find out which foods or lifestyle habits can trigger an episode.
- Two per cent of the population suffer from food allergies, and up to 40 per cent suffer from a form of food intolerance.

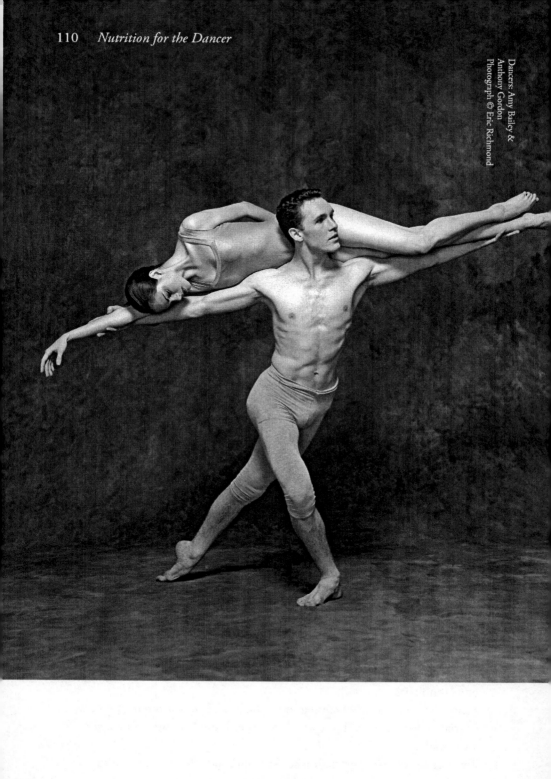

Chapter 11
Dance and Osteoporosis

> *In a dancer, there is a reverence for such forgotten things as the miracle of the small beautiful bones and their delicate strength.*
>
> **Martha Graham**

Osteoporosis: an unfamiliar word for many young dancers, despite its immeasurable threat to a talented career.

It is a 'silent epidemic' that many do not realise they are suffering from until they fracture a bone by the simplest of movements. Once characterised as a bone disorder suffered by women over the age of fifty, osteoporosis is increasing at an alarming rate among young women in their twenties, with serious signs of weak and brittle bones appearing. Even more worrying is the group of individuals who are most likely to develop a bone disorder that can devastate aspirations of a life on stage: dancers. And even though injury can destroy hopes of maintaining a long-term successful career, the 'at any cost' attitude that so many young and talented dancers have means that they place health second to their quest for a slender figure. Is there any point in having the perfect physique if you cannot use it?

Quite simply, osteoporosis is a preventable disorder, and avoiding it does not mean one cannot maintain an ideal physique. Health professionals, teachers and parents, by providing valuable advice and support, are thus vitally important to budding young dancers making their way in the world of dance.

What is osteoporosis?

One or more of several factors can contribute to the development of vulnerable bones. The word 'osteoporosis' literally means 'porous bones', reflecting the thinning and deterioration of bone when minerals stored in its structure are leached out for other purposes. Bones store a vast number of minerals, particularly calcium, potassium, zinc, phosphorus and magnesium.

A healthy skeleton constantly repairs and rebuilds itself in order to support the body. Old bone is broken down and replaced with new, stronger bone – an activity controlled and influenced by hormones, exercise and nutrition.

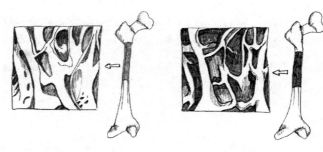

Figure 10. Healthy bone   Figure 11. Osteoporosis

When bone is depleted of minerals and other components that make up its structure, the volume of bone mass decreases. This creates large crevices that reduce the bones' ability to withstand the pressure of muscles pulling on them during dance. When stress placed on the skeleton becomes too much, bones can fracture.

Bone deterioration in dancers is exceptionally difficult to diagnose in its early stages, as it only emerges as pain, discomfort or a fracture. Only when a bone scan is performed can weak and brittle bones be diagnosed.

What causes osteoporosis?

When minerals, hormones and other components making up the body's chemistry are present in the correct amounts, the body is 'in balance'. When this balance is disrupted, minerals change their behaviour in relation to each other and do not function correctly or do their job adequately. Factors that influence this careful balance are nutrition, hormones and exercise.

Nutrition

Many dancers compromise their food intake either by consuming foods of little value (such as fast food or confectionery) or by consuming too few calories.

Dancers restricting their food intake are most likely to cut back on foods that happen to be rich sources of two important components for healthy bone: calcium and protein. Smoking and excessive amounts of caffeine and alcohol also have a negative effect on bone.

Calcium is a very important mineral for healthy bones, and if the diet fails to provide adequate amounts of it, the body is forced to sacrifice its stores to make sure there is enough calcium in the bloodstream. Low-fat dairy foods are ideal for dancers, as they contain just as much calcium as full-fat dairy products and are also a good source of other vitamins, minerals and high-quality protein. Including two to four portions of low-fat dairy foods will provide the right amount of calcium. Fish, fortified soya products and breakfast cereals also contain good amounts of calcium.

Protein is another important factor in the absorption of calcium, and a lack of it can make the dancer more susceptible to fractures. Low-protein diets can also cause muscles to become weak, so that bones move out of alignment and become more vulnerable to injury. Two to four portions of protein-rich foods each day will ensure an adequate protein intake.

An excess of phosphorus (found in fizzy drinks) can also lead to thinning bones, because large quantities of it can leach calcium from bone. Choosing alternative fluids such as squashes, water, fruit juice and cordials will greatly reduce the amount of phosphorus in the diet if you find you are consuming too much.

Fruit and vegetables provide a good source of vitamins and minerals, particularly vitamin C and vitamin D, which both play an important role in the growth, maintenance and repair of bone. The major source of vitamin D is from sunlight on our skin, but food sources include oily fish, eggs and fortified cereals. Low exposure to the sun during winter months, combined with a diet lacking in vitamin D, could lead to a deficiency of this vitamin and to abnormal skeletal growth. Vitamin C deficiency slows down the healing and repair of bone. Five portions of fruit and vegetables in the diet each day will supply an abundance of vitamins and minerals and will also help to keep a dancer trim.

Healthy fats (such as olive oil and oily fish) also increase the absorption of calcium in the intestine, and only small amounts of healthy oils are required to achieve this.

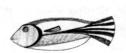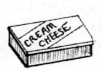

Hormones

When energy output (energy burnt off each day) does not match energy consumed in the form of calories, our body's natural balance is disrupted, and hormones in particular suffer in consequence. One such hormone is oestrogen, the female sex hormone. Low body weight, low fat percentage, inadequate calorie intake, an imbalanced diet and smoking can all contribute to low circulating levels of oestrogen, which is the number one hormone for healthy bones in women.

Together with the hormone progesterone, oestrogen controls the female reproductive system, including body shape and fertility, and insufficient levels of oestrogen can lead the menstrual cycle to become irregular or stop completely. Although the convenience of this may appeal to many young dancers, the lack of menstrual periods (amenorrhoea) has long-term health implications, particularly for bone. Oestrogen deficiency affects the careful balance of bone maintenance, whereby more bone is broken down than is being replaced. This causes bones to become weak, brittle and more vulnerable to fracture. Sudden weight loss and psychological stress are also linked to loss of menstruation.

A lack of menstrual periods is simply the body's way of slowing or shutting down its normal running in order to minimise the loss of energy. In this case it has shut down fertility, in that the dancer is no longer fertile. This has a devastating effect on healthy bones. Fortunately, a healthy diet and lifestyle can reverse this effect, so that menstruation can return and bones do not suffer.

Exercise

Weight-bearing exercise has a positive effect on bone and can decrease the risk of osteoporosis. This is because bones, reacting to avoid fracture, strengthen when muscles attached to them exert a force or pulling motion. Weight-bearing exercise includes brisk walking and dancing (note, though, that ballet dancing is predominately non-weight-bearing), tennis, aerobics and using light weights. Any form of exercise where you are supporting the weight of your body (such as jumping or skipping) is recognised as weight-bearing.

Some dancers suffer from amenorrhoea due to the amount of stress over-training places on the body. Although loss of menstruation is unlikely to occur as a result of exercise alone, it can often be brought on by a number of factors, such as restricted eating, high-intensity training, low body fat, and physical or mental stress.

Young dancers who undertake intensive training before puberty may also experience a delay in menstruation, as physical stress placed on the body can affect hormones involved in the development of the female physique. This can put such dancers at slighter greater risk of osteoporosis in later life.

Summary

- Osteoporosis, a preventable disorder, is a 'silent epidemic' that many are unaware they suffer from until they break a bone doing the simplest of movements.
- An alarming number of young dancers now show signs of weak, porous bones with a bone density comparable to that of women over the age of 50.
- Many factors contribute to the prevalence of osteoporosis, including exercise, nutrition and hormone balance.
- Calcium, vitamin C, vitamin D and protein are necessary for strong bones, and phosphorus found in fizzy drinks has a negative effect on bone density.
- Low circulating oestrogen levels in women are associated with an increased risk of osteoporosis. Those most at risk are dancers suffering from a lack of menstrual periods (amenorrhoea).
- Weight-bearing exercise has been shown to have a positive effect on bone density.

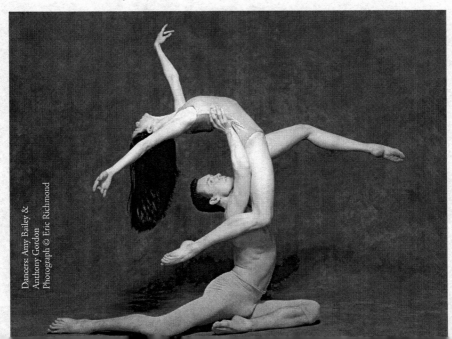

Dancers: Amy Bailey & Anthony Gordon
Photograph © Eric Richmond

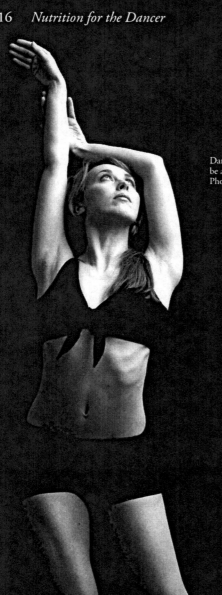

Dancer: Emily McElligott 'Having a good diet means that I will
be able to dance for longer, which is ultimately what I love to do!'
Photograph © Cassie Moore: AM-London

Chapter 12
Injury, Nutrition and Recovery

Dancing should look easy; like an optical illusion. It should seem effortless. When you do a difficult variation, the audience is aware that it is demanding and that you have the power and strength to do it. But in the end, when you take your bow, you should look as if you were saying, 'Oh, it was nothing. I could do it again.'

Bruce Marks

Across all professions within society, the human body is most challenged through dance, exploring what the body can achieve under immense stress: stress that comes from performing on stage, physical stress from years of intense training, competitive stress during countless auditions, stress associated with maintaining the necessary body shape, stress coping with an injury, and stress to surpass oneself artistically and skilfully. Performance nerves, anxiety, financial stress, late nights, immense fatigue, and stress upon retirement from stage: one cannot underestimate the huge accomplishment of a dancer who succeeds within this performing art.

Dealing with an injury is an immense challenge for a dancer; encouraging insufferable bouts of anxiety in relation to future stage aspirations and financial frustrations. But the most crucial step towards surviving with – and preventing – an injury, is finding the cause – and the right one. Poor technique, over-exercising, low bone mineral density, fatigue, low body weight, low fat percentage, inadequate calorie intake and poor food choice all predispose a dancer to injury. A dancer must recognise the culprit, or combination of culprits, that have made them vulnerable to injury, and then take positive steps towards correcting the situation. The self-assurance, confidence and positivity that accompanies a dancer's decision to take control is immeasurably self-empowering – the mind has committed the person, and the body can only follow.

Injury during training or performance may happen at some point in a dancer's career: an unfortunate fact of life. Sprains, muscle tears, fractures, bruises and the occasional cuts and abrasions are common occurrences, and will need nutrients well over and above the usual requirements in order to replace damaged cells with spanking new ones. When faced with inadequate supplies of vital, high-quality nutrients, the body will be forced to hunt around in search of the odd stray nutrient in an attempt to help the injured party recover. It will have to make the best of a bad situation. Alternatively, an injured body can get back on the road to recovery, and cause far fewer problems, if it has been offered crucial supplies.

A helping hand

The first step on the road to recovery is that the injury will become inflamed, painful, red and hot. All of these uncomfortable and inconvenient responses promote the same thing – a good supply of blood, rich with white blood cells, proteins, nutrients and a host of other substances that will guarantee optimal healing. The key nutrients involved in recovery include protein, vitamin C, zinc, iron, vitamin A, vitamin B complex, vitamin E and selenium. Calcium and vitamin D play chief roles in the healing of bone tissue.

Maintaining your strength and, at the same time, minimising any gain in weight will also be a criterion. Being confident that the foods you choose are not contributing to weight gain is an incredibly important step towards recovery, and a nutrient-rich but low-fat diet will overcome the difficulty of getting back into shape after an injury and will also ensure that injured cells are replaced with healthy cells.

Protein

Protein is absolutely vital for the healing of connective tissue, ligaments and bone. Moreover, it has been shown that a diet low in protein can have a detrimental effect on recovery time and on the quality of new tissue that replaces damaged tissue. After water, protein is the most abundant substance in the human body, and particularly so for dancers. Rich sources of protein include lean poultry, lean red meat, fish, eggs, low-fat dairy products, quorn, soya products, beans and pulses. Aim to fill a third of your plate or a third of your lunch and main meal with a good source of protein (see Chapter 3 for more on protein).

Vitamin C

Vitamin C plays a leading role in the formation of new collagen, the main component in connective tissue and ligaments. It activates the enzyme responsible for making new collagen, and adds tensile strength to new tissue, allowing it to stretch without tearing. Vitamin C also increases the activity of white blood cells and their recruitment to an injury, clearing away damaged cells to make room for the formation of new scar tissue. A lack of vitamin C delays healing time because new scar tissue is then too fragile and cannot be formed adequately.

Vitamin C is found in all fruits and vegetables, particularly in citrus fruits, juices, strawberries, tomatoes, broccoli, sweet and white potatoes and cantaloupe. Other excellent sources include papaya, mango, watermelon, Brussels sprouts, cauliflower, cabbage, winter squash, red peppers, raspberries, blueberries, cranberries and pineapples.

Zinc

Zinc is crucial for healing, forming part of the structure in more than 200 important enzymes that are at the forefront of cell growth and repair. Zinc deficiency is quite common amongst dancers; if this is true in your case, ensuring that you include rich sources of zinc in your diet will speed up the healing process.

Good sources of zinc include lean meat, fish, shellfish, pulses, seeds, nuts and wholegrains.

Calcium and vitamin D

Calcium is particularly important when an injury involves bone tissue. Bone is essentially a protein matrix or frame within which calcium salts are deposited, making bone strong, flexible and able to withstand the pulling force from muscles attached to it. Vitamin D is needed for the absorption of calcium from the digestive system. Phosphate and magnesium are also present in this matrix.

Rich sources of calcium include low-fat dairy foods, green leafy vegetables, canned sardines, canned mackerel in tomato sauce, canned salmon (flesh and bone), tofu, nuts, sesame and sunflower seeds and dried figs. Your skin can make vitamin D from sunlight, which is the major source of this vitamin. Foods high in vitamin D include oily fish, fish liver oil, egg yolk and fortified margarine.

Preventing weight gain

An injury will temporarily enforce the suspension of training and performance to a greater or lesser extent, so during this time the diet must encourage the injury to heal whilst preventing the dancer from gaining weight. Chapter 1 showed you how to calculate your resting metabolic rate, which tells you how many calories you need without any form of movement (so, lying down but not sleeping). Calculating your daily energy expenditure then tells you how many calories you require for everyday movement (walking to and from work, shopping etc). When you have an injury, and are doing less exercise, this is how much you should aim to eat each day – with a few minor changes!

You will need just as much lean protein as before; but now that you are not exercising as much, you do not need quite as much carbohydrate. This may simply mean fewer starchy snacks, or you may just need a little less carbohydrate with your usual meals. The 'third of a plate rule' still applies, whereby a third of your plate (or a third of your meal) should be filled with lean protein, a third with carbohydrate and a third with salad/vegetables/fruit. To help control appetite, and make you feel satisfied after a meal, you may want to increase the quantity of salad and vegetables on your plate: these are naturally low in calories and full of nutrients. Do make sure you still include something starchy, such as rice or potatoes. If you cut back too much, you will feel lethargic and lack strength – which you can't afford to do.

As far as possible, try to avoid foods high in fat, particularly unhealthy saturated fat (for a full description, refer to Chapter 4). This will certainly help you to keep trim while you are not training as intensively. Healthy oils found in oily fish, nuts and seeds are important for healing and reducing inflammation, and therefore including one or two portions of oily fish per week, or snacking on a small handful of nuts and seeds, will ensure you are getting your omegas!

Table 12.1 gives you more information on what sort of things you should be eating.

Table 12.1. Foods to eat during recovery from an injury

Grains & cereals

Eat every day

Wholegrain flour, bread, crispbread, brown rice and wholemeal pasta, potatoes, wholegrain breakfast cereals (wheat- or bran-based, porridge)

Take in moderate amounts (every few days)
Refined white flour, white bread, rice, refined cereals (rice-based, cornflakes)
Low-fat oven chips, roasted potatoes

Leave on the shelf, or have as a treat
Pastries, fried rice, pasta in creamy sauces
Sugar- or honey-coated cereals
Chips and fried potatoes

Fruit & vegetables

Eat every day
Fresh, frozen or tinned (in own juice)

Take in moderate amounts (every few days)
Fruit with sugar

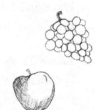

Leave on the shelf, or have as a treat
Fruit with cream!

Protein

Eat every day
Lean chicken, white fish, shellfish, beans and lentils, quorn, tofu

Take in moderate amounts (every few days)
Oily fish, fish paste, smoked fish, low-fat sausages, eggs, lean red meat

Leave on the shelf, or have as a treat
Prepared meal products, sausages, pâté, streaky bacon, salami meat pies, fatty meat, fried meat, fried eggs

Dairy

Eat every day
Low-fat yoghurts, low-fat fromage frais, semi-skimmed/skimmed milk, light cream cheese, cottage cheese

Take in moderate amounts (every few days)
Low-fat polyunsaturated spreads and cheese

Leave on the shelf, or have as a treat
Butter, hard cheese, whole milk, cream, thick & creamy yoghurts, ice cream

Snacks*

Eat every day
Small snacks:
Fruit, vegetable sticks, crispbread with lean meat, low-fat yoghurts, mini-pitta bread, healthy muffin, teacakes, raisin bread, plain biscuits

Take in moderate amounts (every few days)
Moderate-sized snacks:
Handful of dried fruit and nuts, boiled sweets, bagels, bread rolls, pitta bread with healthy fillings

Leave on the shelf, or have as a treat
Cream and cream-filled cakes and biscuits, chocolates, toffees, marzipans, crisps, cheese and crackers

Fluids

Drink every day
Water, fruit and herbal teas, coffee, sugar-free squashes

Take in moderate amounts (every few days)
Pure fruit juices, alcohol, cordials, low-fat milky drinks

Leave on the shelf, or have as a treat
Hot chocolate, full-fat milk lattes

* Increase or decrease snack depending on the amount of exercise undertaken.

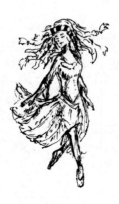

Appendices

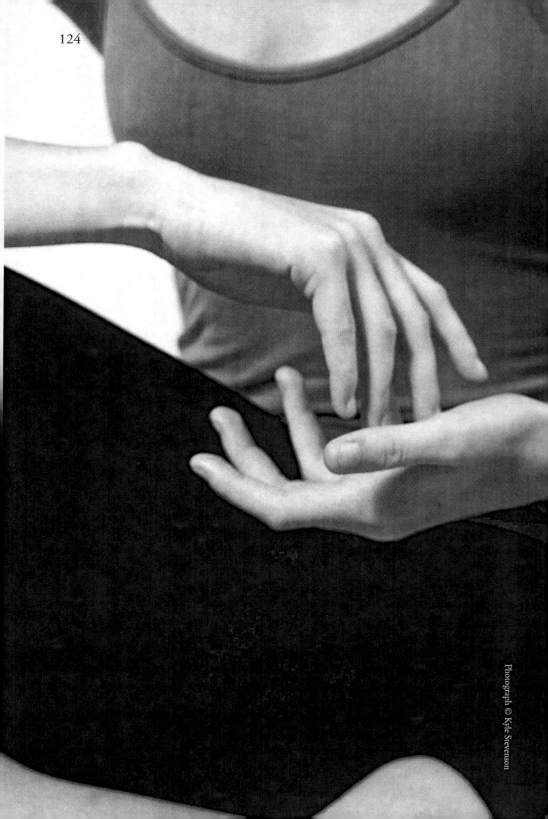

The Dancer's Kitchen

To provide a little inspiration, here are some healthy foods and drinks that are ideal for the dancer's kitchen cupboard, fridge and freezer. Ideas for sandwich fillings and for making sports drinks are listed too.

Stock cupboard ideas

Staples

Pasta: assorted shapes and sizes
Packet rice: long-grain / wild rice / risotto
Couscous
Egg noodles / rice noodles
Potatoes
Oat bran
Flour (to make muffins etc.)
Crispbread / rice cakes / oatcakes / cream crackers
Dried fruit
Tinned fruit in natural juice
Tinned soup

Breakfast cereals

Oats for porridge
Wheat-based cereals
Muesli

Bran flakes
Cornflakes and rice-based cereals (to mix with muesli and bran flakes)

Protein

Tinned salmon
Tinned tuna in brine
Tinned sardines / mackerel / anchovies
Eggs
Tinned and dried pulses
Tinned baked beans

Sauces / dressings / herbs and spices

Salt and pepper
Olive oil and vegetable oil
Stock cubes
Gravy granules
Vinegar
Soy sauce
Tomato ketchup
Chutney
Tomato salsa
Tomato purée
Carton of passata
Lemon juice
Dried mixed herbs
Cinnamon or mixed-spice powder
Ground ginger
Dried mint
chilli powder
Curry powder
Parsley
Baking powder

Drinks

Tea – herbal and fruit
Coffee
Sugar-free cordials and squashes

Foods for the fridge

Low-fat natural/flavoured yoghurt
Low-fat fromage frais
0%-fat Greek-style yoghurt
Reduced-fat cream cheese
Reduced-fat hummus
Tofu pieces
Cottage cheese
Chicken slices
Ham slices
Semi-skimmed/skimmed milk
Fruit (apples, pears and in-season fruit)
Salad (tomatoes, cucumber, lettuce, celery)
Vegetables (carrots, parsnips, onions, mushrooms, broccoli, courgettes,
    cauliflower, peppers, leeks etc.)
Fresh chicken breast
Lean beef mince
Peeled prawns

Freezer foods

Frozen vegetables
Frozen fruit
Plain unbreaded fish fillets (cod / plaice / salmon etc.)
Frozen prawns
Frozen chicken, lean beef mince
Sorbet
Ice cream (for treats)
Sliced bread / rolls / pitta bread / bagels
Home-made frozen meals

Sandwich fillings

Many types of bread are ideal for sandwiches, including wholemeal, multigrain, rye, herb, baguette, ciabatta, bagel, wholemeal pitta and sun-dried tomato breads and rolls.

Choose from one of the following healthy low-fat fillings:

- Chicken slices or pieces, light cream cheese and tomato
- Ham slices, lettuce and tomato
- Reduced-fat hummus with lettuce and cucumber
- Cottage cheese, yeast extract, tomato slices and lettuce
- Tuna, light cream cheese, salt and pepper to season
- Tuna, red kidney beans and tomato sauce
- Turkey and cranberry sauce
- Chicken pieces, sweetcorn and low-fat fromage frais
- Boiled egg, lettuce, tomato and low-fat dressing
- Grated carrot, raisins and apple.

Making sports drinks at home

Hypotonic sports drinks – for fast absorption

Recipe 1
50ml fruit squash (not the sugar-free variety)
450ml plain water
0.5g of salt (optional)

Recipe 2
250ml fruit juice (orange / apple etc.)
750ml water
1g of salt (optional)

Isotonic sports drinks – for hydration and refueling

Recipe 1
100ml fruit squash (not the sugar-free variety)
400ml plain water
0.5g of salt (optional)

Recipe 2
250ml fruit juice (orange / apple etc.)
250ml plain water
0.5g of salt (optional)

The Balanced Diet Explained

The 'third of a plate' rule

The 'third of a plate' rule can be applied to your lunch or evening meal, and is a very good way of ensuring that you're not omitting any nutrients, and that you haven't overindulged.

This rule doesn't incorporate snacks and suitable foods for breakfast; therefore to guarantee that your overall diet is balanced, use the 'third of a plate' rule together with the portion control described in Appendix 3.

A THIRD of your plate or meal should be CARBOHYDRATE:

- e.g. rice, pasta, potatoes, couscous, noodles, spaghetti, sliced bread, baguette, bagels, pitta, crisp bread etc.

A THIRD of your plate or meal should be PROTEIN:

- e.g. chicken, turkey, shellfish, oily fish, white fish, lamb, beef, pork, eggs, dairy, quorn, beans and pulses, nuts

A THIRD of your plate or meal should be SALAD / FRUIT / VEGETABLES.

> **Tip**
> Choose salad, fruits and vegetables of different colours, as each colour represents a different important nutrient.

The eatwell plate

Use the eatwell plate to help you get the balance right. It shows how
much of what you eat should come from each food group.

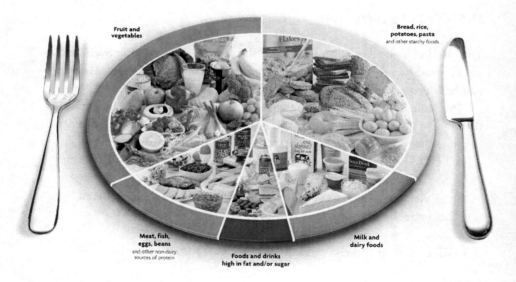

Check the fat content!!

Very importantly, the meal you have just prepared must be low in fat. Here's a check-list for a low-fat meal:

- Avoid processed foods and foods that are breaded, battered or fried. Instead, choose unbreaded chicken and fish, and bake, boil or grill it.
- Avoid creamy-based sauces, and opt for tomato- or stock-based sauces.
- Avoid grating cheese, or adding butter to your meal. Choose a low-fat cream cheese or fromage frais.
- Limit mayonnaise and other high-fat dressings, and choose low-fat alternative such as tomato sauces, soy sauce, brown sauce and chutneys.
- Only add one tablespoon of vegetable oil (olive oil in salads) per person to get the right amount of essential oils.

Variety is the key

The key to a healthy and varied diet is to use different ingredients when cooking. This doesn't mean you need to prepare complicated recipes or have a large stock cupboard. You can be imaginative by simply varying your sources of protein, carbohydrate and dressings.

Carbohydrate

Rather than having pasta every night, for example, alternate it with jacket potatoes, rice, spaghetti, egg noodles, different shapes of pasta, couscous etc. Instead of having sliced bread every day, vary it with bagels, pitta breads, baguettes, rolls and wraps. They are all very similar in calorie content and are all equally low in fat.

Protein

For variety and health, choose chicken once or twice a week, white fish / oily fish / shellfish a few times a week, beans and pulses on another night, and lean red meat (lean mince, for example) once a week. Not only are you following a healthy balanced diet, but you will also enjoy a range of meals.

Dressings and sauces

To jazz up a meal, use a variety of dressings and sauces to complement the meal. Examples include tomato-based sauces, soy sauce, low-fat fromage frais, ginger and lemon, a sprinkle of chilli powder and mango chutney.

Appendix 3
How Many Portions?

A dancer's diet can also be illustrated in terms of the number of portions, and their size. Where possible, aim to spread portions evenly throughout the day to maximise your energy levels and metabolism.

Fruits and vegetables

Choose 5–9 portions of fruit and vegetables each day (3–5 servings of vegetables and 2–4 servings of fruit).

They are rich in vital nutrients essential for a dancer's health and career in performance. Being very low in fat and calories, they are ideal as accompaniments to meals, and make great snacks.

One vegetable portion = 80g, which is about the amount you can fit into the palm of your hand (1 carrot, 2 tablespoons, 2–3 spears of broccoli, 5 cherry tomatoes).

One fruit portion = 80g, which will work out at about the size of a tennis ball (1 apple, 8–10 strawberries, 2 satsumas).

Grains and potatoes

Choose 4–6 portions from this group; one portion is about the size of a clenched fist (for example, 2 slices of bread, 1 bagel, 40–50g of breakfast cereal, 5 tablespoons or 180g of cooked pasta or rice).

This food group is rich in carbohydrate, and provides a source of energy essential for a dancer. Include a breakfast cereal, bread, rice, pasta, spaghetti, noodles or oats with each meal and snack for a steady supply of energy and to maintain stable blood sugars. Choose wholegrain where possible.

Calcium-rich foods

You need a total of 2–4 portions of calcium-rich foods each day (low-fat dairy products, nuts, fish with soft bones or pulses) for healthy bones and contracting muscles.

One portion is equivalent to 1 pot of low-fat yoghurt or fromage frais (150g), 200ml semi / skimmed milk, 200ml soya milk fortified with calcium, matchbox-size portion of tofu or cheese.

Protein-rich foods

Including 2–4 portions of protein rich foods is essential for an active dancer in terms of strength and stamina, developing lean-toned muscles and a healthy metabolism.

One portion of 100g, equivalent in size to a large clenched fist, might consist of 3 thick slices of lean meat, half a small chicken breast, 1 fish fillet, 2 eggs, 5 tablespoons of beans / lentils, or 1–2 soya / quorn sausages. Low-fat dairy products can also be counted as a protein portion.

Healthy fats and oils

Essential oils found in oily fish, nuts, seeds, olive oil, sunflower oil, rapeseed oil and flaxseed oil are absolutely vital for a dancer's joints and immune system, and help in preventing and recovering from injury. In terms of health, these oils help to keep the heart in good health and to prevent cardiovascular disease – important even to the slim dancer!

One portion is equivalent to 1 tablespoon of olive oil / vegetable oil, 2 level tablespoons of nuts and seeds (or a small handful) or 1 oily fish steak (the size of a deck of cards).

Discretionary calories

Being a dancer means that you need a few extra calories to support the demands of a class, rehearsal or performance, and this is over and above the portions specified in the food groups mentioned above.

This can be in the form of an extra snack such as a healthy muffin, a chewy bar or a healthy dessert. And the more classes you take, the more active you are, hence the need for a few more snacks!

Recipes for Snacks and Meals

All the recipes in this appendix are quick to prepare, perfect for the dancer and inexpensive to make. Each is low in fat, provides a balanced source of protein and carbohydrate, and is rich in vitamins and minerals.

Spicy chicken

Serving size: 2   Per serving: 600kcal   50g protein

2 × 150g (5oz) chicken breasts or chicken pieces
175g (6oz) rice
1 onion
green salad or vegetables (lettuce, cucumber, broccoli, green beans etc.)
2 tablespoons vegetable oil
2 crushed garlic cloves
1–2 tablespoons curry powder
2 tablespoons tomato purée
salt and pepper to taste

1. Place the chicken under the grill for approx. 15 mins, turning occasionally.
2. Boil the rice for approx. 20 mins (or follow instructions on the packet).
3. Heat the vegetable oil in a pan, then add the chopped onion and cook until golden (approx. 5 mins).
4. Add the garlic and curry powder and cook for a further 1–2 mins.
5. Remove the chicken from the grill, chop into pieces and add to the pan with the tomato puree and water.
6. Cover and cook for a further 5–10 mins.
7. Serve the spicy chicken with rice and a bed of salad or green vegetables.

Moroccan chicken with couscous

Couscous is quite widely available in the supermarkets, and is a very healthy source of carbohydrate. It requires very little cooking (simply add boiling water!) and produces a light, fluffy accompaniment to meat, fish and vegetables.

Serving size: 2   Per serving: 670kcal   48g protein

2 × 150g (5oz) chicken breasts or chicken pieces
160g (5oz) uncooked couscous
6 chopped dried apricots
200g tinned chickpeas

1 onion
2 tablespoons vegetable oil
2 cloves garlic
1 teaspoon ginger powder
¼ pint (150ml) water

1. Place couscous in a bowl, add 250ml boiled water. Cover and leave.
2. Heat the vegetable oil in a pan, then add the chopped onion, garlic, ginger powder and chicken pieces. Stir-fry for approx. 4–5 mins.
3. Add the chickpeas, apricots and water.
4. Cook on a low heat for 15 mins.
5. Serve chicken on a bed of couscous and lettuce.

Potato and fish pie

Serving size: 2   Per serving: 375kcal   40g protein

450g (1lb) potatoes
200g (8oz) white fish (cod, plaice etc.) or oily fish (tinned salmon, mackerel)
4 tablespoons (50ml) semi-skimmed or skimmed milk
2 eggs
squeeze of lemon juice
1 tablespoon Lemon Thyme

1. Boil the roughly cut potatoes until tender.
2. Drain away the water. Mash, and add milk, beaten eggs, flaked fish parsley and lemon juice.
3. Place all ingredients into a dish and cook for 20 mins at 200°C / 400°F.
4. Serve with a selection of vegetables or salad.

Prawn stir-fry

Serving size: 2   Per serving: 500kcal   35g protein

250g (9oz) frozen or fresh green beans
200g (8oz) frozen or fresh peeled prawns
175g (6oz) egg noodles or tagliatelle

2 tablespoons vegetable oil
1 tablespoon soy sauce

1. Boil noodles (or tagliatelle) for approx.10–15 mins.
2. Boil green beans in boiling water for approx. 5 mins.
3. Whilst noodles and green beans are cooking, heat the vegetable oil in a pan and stir-fry the prawns for 2 mins.
4. Drain beans and noodles then add to prawns and soy sauce.
5. Serve.

Crispy salmon

Serving size: 2   Per serving: 500kcal   33g protein

200g (8oz) tinned salmon
selection of vegetables thickly chopped (carrots, onions, parsnips, broccoli, leeks etc.)
175g (6oz) uncooked egg noodles
1 tablespoon mixed herbs
salt and pepper to season

1. Boil vegetables for 5–10 mins to soften.
2. Drain and place under the grill with the salmon and season with mixed herbs, salt and pepper.
3. Meanwhile, boil egg noodles for 10–15 mins.
4. When vegetables and salmon are crispy, remove from grill and serve on a bed of noodles.

Spicy tuna and jacket potato

Serving size: 2   Per serving: 475 kcal   40g protein

2 medium-sized potatoes (260g each)
200g (8oz) tinned tuna, drained
4 tablespoons red kidney beans
4 tablespoons sweetcorn
splash of Tabasco or chilli sauce

1. Cook jacket potato in microwave (cover in kitchen tissue) or cover in foil and cook in oven for approx. 90 mins.
2. Mix and heat tuna, kidney beans, sweetcorn and Tabasco in a pan.
3. Serve.

Chilli with rice

Serving size: 2   Per serving: 550kcal   32g protein

200g (8oz) lean beef mince
175g (6oz) rice
1 onion
1 carton of passata (300ml)
selection of frozen vegetable mix (peas, carrots etc.)
1 tablespoon of chilli powder
salt and pepper to taste

1. Heat the chopped onion in a little water for 1 min.
2. Add beef mince and stir-fry for a further 2 mins until the meat is browned.
3. Add frozen vegetables, passata and chilli powder and simmer for 15–20 mins.
4. Meanwhile, boil rice in a pan for 15 mins.
5. Serve the chilli on a bed of rice, and add salt and pepper.

Healthy beefburgers

Serving size: 2   Per serving: 325kcal   28g protein

200g (8oz) lean beef mince
2 medium bread rolls / baps
1 onion
1 tablespoon dried mint
salt and pepper to taste

1. Heat the chopped onion in a little water for 1 min.
2. Mix onion, beef mince and mint in a bowl and mould into 2 large burgers. Season with salt and pepper.

3.   Cook for approx. 25 mins at 200°C / 400°F.
4.   Serve burger in a roll or bap with tomato sauce, lettuce and tomato.

Potato omelette

Serving size: 2   Per serving: 475kcal   30g protein

450g (1lb) potatoes
1 tablespoon vegetable oil
1 onion
5 eggs
salt and pepper
paprika

1.   Boil the roughly cut potatoes until tender.
2.   Heat the oil, add the chopped onions and stir-fry for 3 mins.
3.   Beat the eggs, add salt and pepper, and pour into the pan
      with the onions.
4.   Reduce the heat and cook for a further 5 mins, sprinkling
      with paprika.
5.   Serve on a bed of salad.

Tip
To crisp and brown the omelette, place under a grill for a further
1–2 mins.

Mixed bean hotpot

Serving size: 2   Per serving: 550kcal   28g protein

450g (1lb) potatoes, boiled and cooled
400g (14oz) tinned mixed beans (e.g. red kidney beans, chickpeas,
haricot beans)
250g tinned tomatoes
100g (4oz) green beans or red peppers
1 tablespoon tomato purée
1 tablespoon mixed herbs

1. Drain the tinned beans and place in a casserole dish.
2. Add the green beans (or red peppers) with tomatoes, tomato purée and herbs.
3. Thinly slice the potatoes and arrange on top of the mixture.
4. Bake at 200°C / 400°F for approx. 25–30 mins and serve with salad or vegetables.

Vegetable stew

Serving size: 2   Per serving: 400kcal   15g protein

450g (1lb) mixed chunky vegetables (carrots, aubergines,
broad beans, courgettes, mushrooms, parsnips etc.)
175g (6oz) uncooked couscous
150ml (¼ pint) water
1 vegetable stock cube
salt and pepper to season

1. Place couscous in a bowl with 250ml boiled water mixed with the stock cube. Cover and leave.
2. Cook vegetables on a low heat, and simmer until very tender.
3. Serve vegetables on a bed of couscous.

Fruity yoghurt

Serving size: 1   Per serving: 275kcal   18g protein

150g 0%-fat Greek yoghurt or low-fat fromage frais
1 banana
1 apple
¼ tin mixed fruit (cherries, pineapple, grapes etc.)
1 teaspoon sugar
cinnamon or mixed spice

1. Chop all the fruit and mix into a bowl.
2. Spoon in the yoghurt or fromage frais.
3. Lightly dust with sugar and cinnamon and serve chilled.

Healthy oat muffins

Serving size: 10–12 muffins   Per serving: 135kcal   5g protein

250g oat bran
350ml semi-skimmed or skimmed milk
1 tablespoon baking powder
1 teaspoon allspice
50g (2oz) sugar
1 tablespoon vegetable oil
2 egg whites
50g dried fruit (e.g. raisins)

1. Preheat oven to 220°C / 425°F.
2. Mix together oat bran, baking powder, cinnamon and sugar.
3. Add milk, egg whites and dried fruit.
4. Mould into 10–12 muffins (preferably have some paper cases or bun tins to hand, otherwise shape muffins and place them on a tin tray into the oven).
5. Bake for approx. 10–15 mins.

Tasty chewy bars

Serving size: 15 bars   Per serving: 115kcal   5g protein

250g (9 fl oz) low-fat natural yoghurt
250g (9oz) low-fat soft cheese
100g (4oz) dried fruit
50g (2oz) margarine
3 tablespoons honey
75g (3oz) muesli
75g (3oz) self-raising flour
2 eggs

1. Mix together margarine and honey.
2. Mix in remaining ingredients.
3. Spoon mixture into a baking tin greased with a little margarine.
4. Bake for 20 mins or until firm and browned.
5. Slice into 15 bars and serve warm or chilled.

Spicy baked apples

Serving size: 1   Per serving: 215kcal   10g protein

1 large cooking apple
1 tablespoon dried fruit (raisins, sultanas etc.)
1 teaspoon sugar or honey
cinnamon or mixed spice
150g natural low-fat yoghurt or low-fat fromage frais or low-fat custard

1.   Remove core from apple.
2.   Lightly pierce the skin, place apple in a small dish.
3.   Fill centre of apple with dried fruit.
4.   Cover with foil and bake at 200°C / 400°F for 40–45 mins.
5.   Serve with yoghurt and cinnamon, fromage frais or custard.

Food Diary Examples

The following menus are simple examples aimed to give dancers a little guidance on planning a balanced diet.

Table A5.1. Menu 1: 1750kcal

	Calories (kcal)	Protein (g)
Breakfast		
1 cup porridge oats (60g)	215	7
300ml skimmed milk / unsweetened soya milk	100	10
1 tablespoon raisins	80	1
Sprinkle of cinnamon / mixed spice	0	0
Mid-morning		
1 home-made chewy bar	115	5
Glass of fruit juice (150ml)	80	0
Lunch		
1 bagel	240	6
Thin layer low-fat cream cheese	20	2
4 chicken slices	100	20
Sliced tomato and lettuce	10	0
Healthy muffin	135	5
Mid-afternoon		
Banana	80	1
Low-fat natural/fruit yoghurt	135	5
Dinner		
1 portion (100g) oily fish	140	20
(tinned mackerel / salmon), lightly grilled		

1 portion mashed potato (3 egg-sized potatoes)	200	8
1 portion mashed carrot (80g)	25	1
1 portion broccoli	25	3
Evening		
1 fruit portion	55	1
TOTAL	**1750kcal**	**95g**

Table A5.2. Menu 2: 1800kcal

	Calories (kcal)	Protein (g)
Breakfast		
2 slices wholemeal toast	175	8
2 level teaspoons jam	50	0
1 pot low-fat fruit yoghurt	135	5
Mid-morning		
1 home-made chewy bar	115	5
1 apple	55	0
Lunch		
1 medium baked potato	200	4
1 portion of tuna in brine (100g)	115	22
in tomato-based sauce		
1 portion of sweetcorn (80g)	80	2
Mid-afternoon		
3 rice cakes	75	2
Low-fat cream cheese (100g)	120	8
Slices of cucumber and tomato	20	0
Low-fat natural / fruit yoghurt	135	5
Dinner		
1 portion chicken (approx. 100g)	120	22
⅓ plate of couscous (80g uncooked)	280	5
1 portion broccoli	30	1
Evening		
1 slice wholemeal toast with small serving of jam	90	4
TOTAL	**1800kcal**	**93g**

Tip
If there are no healthy options or fillings when eating out, try purchasing one part of the meal (e.g. plain baked potato) and bringing your own filling that you have prepared at home.

Table A5.3. Menu 3: 1800kcal

	Calories (kcal)	Protein (g)
Breakfast		
2 slices wholemeal toast	175	8
2 scrambled/poached eggs	170	14
2 teaspoons (10g) olive oil spread	70	0
Mid-morning		
1 pot low-fat natural/fruit yoghurt	135	5
1 banana	80	1
Lunch		
1 large wholemeal pitta	165	7
Half carton (125g) cottage cheese	160	16
1 teaspoon yeast extract (optional!)	10	0
Sliced tomatoes, cucumber and lettuce	10	0
Mid-afternoon		
Healthy muffin	135	5
1 apple	55	0
Dinner		
1 fillet grilled white fish	120	25
2 medium sweet potatoes (300g)	250	4
2 tablespoons low-fat dressing	30	1
1 portion carrots	30	1
1 portion courgettes	30	1
Evening		
1 slice wholemeal toast with light cream cheese	120	6
1 fruit portion	55	1
TOTAL	**1800kcal**	**95g**

Table A5.4. Menu 4 (vegetarian): 1850kcal

	Calories (kcal)	Protein (g)
Breakfast		
2 Shredded Wheat or equivalent (50g)	160	6
200ml skimmed milk	70	7
2 tablespoons (60g) raisins	160	1
Mid-morning		
1 home-made chewy bar	115	5
Lunch		
1 portion noodles (80g uncooked)	280	9
1 portion quorn pieces (4 tablespoon or 100g)	90	12

1 portion sweetcorn (80g)	80	5
1 portion peas (80g)	60	5
Mid-afternoon		
2 rice cakes	50	2
3 tablespoons low-fat cream cheese	100	8
Slices of cucumber and tomato	10	0
Low-fat natural/fruit yoghurt	135	5
Dinner		
1 beanburger	175	11
3 egg-size potatoes	250	4
1 portion carrots	30	1
1 portion courgettes	30	1
Evening		
1 fruit portion	55	1
TOTAL	**1850kcal**	**83g**

Table A5.5. Menu 5: 2150kcal

	Calories (kcal)	Protein (g)
Breakfast		
2 slices wholemeal toast	175	8
2 level teaspoons olive spread	70	0
2 level teaspoons honey	60	0
1 pot low-fat fruit yoghurt	135	5
Mid-morning		
1 home-made chewy bar	115	5
1 large banana	100	1
Lunch		
Pasta salad made with:		
100g pasta	350	10
100g tinned tuna in brine	100	21
Splash of soy sauce	5	0
Chopped red peppers (80g)	20	1
1 glass of orange juice (150ml)	75	1
Mid-afternoon		
3 rice cakes	75	2
3 tablespoons low-fat hummus	100	5
Cucumber slices	10	0

Dinner

1 portion grilled chicken, chopped (150g)	170	30
1 portion rice (100g uncooked)	350	9
1 portion red pepper	20	1
1 portion broccoli	30	3

Evening

1 fruit portion	55	1
1 low-fat fruit yoghurt	135	5

TOTAL	**2150kcal**	**108g**

Table A5.6. Menu 6: 2150kcal

	Calories (kcal)	Protein (g)
Breakfast		
1 bowl muesli (60g)	220	6
1 pot (150g) low-fat natural yoghurt	130	6
/ low-fat fromage frais		
1 tsp honey	35	0
1 glass orange juice (150ml)	75	0
Mid-morning		
1 banana	100	1
1 cereal bar	135	5
Lunch		
1 large roll / bap	300	6
4 slices turkey / chicken	140	22
Lettuce, tomato, cucumber	20	0
1 tablespoon low-fat dressing (chutney,	30	1
tomato salsa, cranberry sauce, cream cheese)		
1 apple	55	1
Mid-afternoon		
Pot of low-fat natural / fruit yoghurt	135	5
2 rice cakes	50	1
Dinner		
⅓ plate tagliatelle (100g uncooked weight)	350	4
100g mixed seafood	120	21
(peeled prawns, haddock, cod etc.)		
50g mushrooms	20	1
1 small onion	20	0
Sauce (15 g flour and 100ml semi-skimmed milk) 35		4

Evening

1 fruit portion	55	1
1 slice wholemeal toast	90	4
1 tablespoon jam	30	0
TOTAL	**2150kcal**	**89g**

Table A5.7. Menu 7: 2150kcal

	Calories (kcal)	Protein (g)
Breakfast		
2 slices wholemeal toast	175	8
2 grilled tomatoes	60	1
2 scrambled/poached eggs	170	14
1 teaspoon olive oil spread	70	0
1 glass of orange juice (150ml)	75	1
Mid-morning		
1 pot low-fat natural/fruit yoghurt	135	5
1 apple	55	1
Lunch		
Couscous (100g uncooked)	350	8
½ tin of mixed beans in spicy tomato sauce	170	11
Small salad	30	1
Mid-afternoon		
Healthy muffin	135	5
Dinner		
Chilli with rice (see recipe)	550	32
Evening		
1 low-fat fruit yoghurt	135	5
1 serving berries	40	1
TOTAL	**2150kcal**	**93g**

Table A5.8. Menu 8: 2100kcal (vegetarian)

	Calories (kcal)	Protein (g)
Breakfast		
1 cup porridge oats (60g)	215	7
300ml skimmed milk / unsweetened soya milk	100	10

1 tablespoon raisins (30g)	85	2
Sprinkle of mixed spice / cinnamon		
1 glass of orange juice	75	1
Mid-morning		
1 home-made chewy bar	115	5
1 large banana	100	1
Lunch		
1 plain tortilla / pitta bread	220	4
½ tin mixed spicy beans with peppers	170	12
Sliced lettuce	20	1
1 low-fat natural/fruit yoghurt	135	5
Mid-afternoon		
4 rice cakes	100	3
3 tablespoons low-fat cream cheese	100	8
Slices of cucumber and tomato	20	1
Dinner		
Potato omelette (see recipe)	475	30
Evening		
1 fruit portion	55	1
1 low-fat fruit yoghurt	135	5
TOTAL	**2100kcal**	**96g**

Table A5.9. Menu 9: 2600kcal

	Calories (kcal)	Protein (g)
Breakfast		
1 small portion muesli mixed with small portion rice snaps (total 70g)	240	5
200ml skimmed milk	70	7
2 slices wholemeal toast	175	8
2 teaspoons olive oil spread	70	0
2 teaspoons jam	70	1
Mid-morning		
1 healthy muffin	135	5
1 large banana	100	1
Lunch		
1 medium baked potato (approx. 320g)	250	5
1 portion chicken pieces (100g) in tomato-based sauce	140	21

1 vegetable portion (80g)	30	1
1 cereal bar	150	3
Mid-afternoon		
4 rice cakes	105	4
100g low-fat hummus	140	8
Slices of cucumber and tomato	10	1
Low-fat natural/fruit yoghurt	135	5
Dinner		
1 fillet grilled flaky white fish	120	22
Lemon juice and black pepper	40	1
(or alternative low-fat dressing)		
2 large sweet potatoes (350g)	400	6
1 portion broccoli	35	3
1 portion carrots	35	1
Evening		
2 slices wholemeal bread	90	4
Thin layer light cream cheese	30	3
TOTAL	**2600kcal**	**115g**

Table A5.10. Menu 10: 2600kcal

	Calories (kcal)	Protein (g)
Breakfast		
Cup of porridge oats (60g)	215	7
300ml skimmed milk	100	10
2 tablespoons raisins (60g)	170	4
1 glass of orange juice	75	1
Mid-morning		
Healthy muffin	135	5
1 fruit portion (apple / pear)	55	1
Lunch		
2 bagels	500	9
3 thick chicken/turkey slices	120	18
2 tablespoons low-fat cream cheese	60	4
Sliced tomato	10	0
Small salad with low-fat dressing	50	1
Mid-afternoon		
Low-fat natural/fruit yoghurt	135	5
Cereal bar	150	4

Dinner

100g (uncooked) pasta	350	10
1 small tin tuna in brine (100g)	115	21
Tomato-based sauce	40	0
2 tablespoons mixed spicy beans (60g)	70	7
1 portion vegetables	60	2

Evening

1 low-fat natural/fruit yoghurt	135	5
1 fruit portion	55	1

TOTAL **2600kcal** **115g**

Table A5.11. Menu 11: 2600kcal

	Calories (kcal)	Protein (g)
Breakfast		
3 slices wholemeal toast	240	12
2 teaspoons olive spread	140	0
3 level teaspoons jam	105	1
1 pot low-fat fruit yoghurt	135	5
Mid-morning		
1 home-made chewy bar	115	5
1 large banana	100	1
Lunch		
1 medium baguette	300	6
Small tin tuna in brine (100g)	115	22
3 tablespoons low-fat cream cheese	100	8
Small salad	50	1
1 apple / pear	55	1
Mid-afternoon		
4 rice cakes	100	4
4 tablespoons low-fat hummus	160	12
Slices of cucumber and tomato	10	0
1 pot low-fat natural/fruit yoghurt	135	5
Dinner		
1 portion chicken, chopped (approx. 150g)	180	35
⅓ plate egg noodles (100g uncooked weight)	390	12
1 portion broccoli	30	3
1 portion carrots	30	1
Soy sauce	0	0

Evening

	Calories (kcal)	Protein (g)
1 jelly pot	105	1
TOTAL	**2600kcal**	**135g**

Table A5.12. Menu 12: 2500kcal (vegetarian)

	Calories (kcal)	Protein (g)
Breakfast		
3 Shredded Wheat or equivalent (70g)	230	7
200ml skimmed milk	70	7
2 tablespoons raisins (60g)	170	4
1 slice wholemeal bread	90	4
1 teaspoon olive spread	70	0
1 teaspoon jam	30	0
1 glass of orange juice (150ml)	75	1
Mid-morning		
1 home-made chewy bar	115	5
1 large banana	100	1
Lunch		
Potato salad made with:		
3 egg-sized potatoes chopped into small pieces (350g)	250	6
Passata / chopped tomatoes	60	2
Portion of tofu cubes (150g)	115	8
Soy sauce	10	0
Small handful chopped green beans	40	1
Lettuce leaves	10	1
1 healthy muffin	135	5
Mid-afternoon		
1 low-fat yoghurt	135	5
1 apple / pear	55	1
Dinner		
⅓ plate portion of rice (100g uncooked)	350	7
½ tin mixed beans in tomato sauce	170	12
2 portions chopped red and green peppers (160g)	60	2
Evening		
1 low-fat yoghurt with berries	160	6
TOTAL	**2500 kcal**	**85g**

Glossary of Vitamins and Minerals

Vitamin	A
Function	Plays a crucial role in helping the body's natural defences fight against viruses and bacteria. Membranes that line the mouth, nose and digestive system rely on vitamin A to perform vital functions. Also an important vitamin for good vision.
	May help treat skin conditions such as acne, eczema and dry skin.
Food sources	Liver, eggs, oily fish, milk, yoghurt, cheese and fortified margarine.
	The body can convert beta-carotene to vitamin A, and food sources of beta-carotene include sweet potatoes, carrots, spinach and dried apricots.
Daily requirements	0.7mg / day for men, and 0.6g / day for women.
Dangers of high doses	Symptoms include headaches, nausea, itchy skin, hair loss and bone deformities. Pregnant women should avoid liver. Limit intake to less than 1.5mg per day.
Those at risk of deficiency	Dancers following a low-fat diet. Vitamin A is fat-soluble, therefore can only be absorbed

if the diet includes small amounts of healthy fat (olive oil, vegetable oil, oily fish, nuts, seeds etc.)

Vitamin	B1 (thiamine)
Function	Important for breaking down carbohydrate for energy, metabolism and proper functioning of muscles, nerves and brain.
Food sources	Wholegrain cereals, potatoes, red meat, milk and dairy products, pulses.
Daily requirements	0.5–0.7mg / day for children, 1mg / day for men, 0.8mg / day for women.
Dangers of high doses	Unlikely to be toxic, as thiamine is water-soluble and any excess is excreted in the urine. Avoid taking more than 3g / day
Those at risk of deficiency	Most common cause of deficiency includes excessive amounts of alcohol, caffeine and smoking. Processed foods tend to be low in B vitamins, and those on a low-calorie or restrictive diet may be more at risk. Symptoms include fatigue and muscle loss.

Vitamin	B2 (riboflavin)
Function	Important for the conversion of carbohydrate into energy. Healthy skin, hair and nails also require adequate amounts of vitamin B2.
Food sources	Yeast and yeast extracts, liver and offal meats, green leafy vegetables, milk and dairy products, meat and meat products.
Daily requirements	0.6–1mg / day for children, 1.3mg / day for men and 1.1mg / day for women.
Dangers of high doses	Most unlikely to be toxic, as any excess is excreted in the urine (visible through its bright yellow colour).
Those at risk of deficiency	Deficiencies can lead to cracks and sores around the nose and mouth.

Vitamin	B3 (niacin)
Function	Important for the conversion of carbohydrate into energy. Healthy skin, nerves and digestive system also require adequate amounts of vitamin B3.
Food sources	Good sources include meat, fish, wholegrain and fortified cereals and milk.
Daily requirements	8–12mg / day for children, 17mg / day for men, 13mg / day for women.
Dangers of high doses	Excess is excreted in the urine, although doses higher than 200mg can cause hot flushes.
Those at risk of deficiency	Deficiency is unlikely in the UK. Severe deficiency seen in deprived populations causes pellagra (lesions in skin exposed to sunlight).

Vitamin	B5 (pantothenic acid)
Function	Important for the metabolism of fats, proteins and carbohydrates. Vitamin B5 also plays a crucial role in fighting infections and in the production of anti-stress hormones.
Food sources	Very widely distributed by food sources that include liver, salmon, tofu, nuts, pulses, eggs and vegetables.
Daily requirements	No daily requirement has been defined.
Dangers of high doses	Excess is excreted in the urine.
Those at risk of deficiency	No deficiency symptoms have been established.

Vitamin	B6 (pyridoxine)
Function	Important for the metabolism of fats, proteins and carbohydrates. Vitamin B6 encourages healthy skin and hair, and is involved in the formation of red blood cells.
Food sources	Pork, chicken, turkey, eggs, bread, wholegrain cereal, potatoes, nuts, pulses and bananas.
Daily requirements	0.7–1mg / day for children, 1.4mg / day for men, 1.2mg / day for women.
Dangers of high doses	Excess is excreted in the urine. However, intakes over 200mg / day over a period of time could lead to neurological problems such as

numbness, and inflammation of the nerves.
Avoid taking over 10mg / day.

Those at risk of deficiency   Clinical deficiency is rare.

Vitamin	B7 (biotin)
Function	Required for the breakdown of protein, fat and carbohydrate into usable energy. Biotin is also vital for the synthesis of fatty acids.
Food sources	Found in many foods, but good sources include kidney and liver, eggs and wholegrain cereals, and it is widely distributed in nuts and seeds.
Daily requirements	No daily requirement has been defined.
Dangers of high doses	No known cases of biotin toxicity.
Those at risk of deficiency	Deficiency is unlikely to occur, but there is a greater risk of it when following a low-calorie or restrictive diet.

Vitamin	B9 (folic acid)
Function	Crucial for the formation of red blood cells and the development of the baby's spine during the first 3 months of pregnancy. Folic acid also plays a key role in preventing heart disease.
Food sources	Found in a wide variety of foods, with good sources being liver and offal, lamb, Brussels sprouts, green vegetables, breakfast cereals and pulses.
Daily requirements	0.07–0.15mg / day for children and 0.2mg / day for adults.
Dangers of high doses	Risk of toxicity is very minimal. High doses may reduce the absorption of zinc and disguise vitamin B12 deficiency.
Those at risk of deficiency	Alcohol, the contraceptive pill and aspirin can reduce the absorption of folic acid. Symptoms include anaemia (resulting in excessive tiredness) and heart disease.

Vitamin	**B12 (cyanocobalamin)**
Function	Vital for the formation of red blood cells and prevention of pernicious anaemia. Also very important for the protection of nerves in the body (it forms part of their protective sheath) and for the absorption of folic acid.
Food sources	Found naturally only in animal food sources: meat and meat products, fish and fish products, and eggs.
	Other sources include fortified vegan foods (such as soya protein and milk), yeast extracts and breakfast cereals (many of which have been fortified with B12).
Daily requirements	Adults need 0.0015mg / day.
Dangers of high doses	Excess is excreted in the urine. Taking 2mg or less is unlikely to cause any harm.
Those at risk of deficiency	Excessive amounts of alcohol and the contraceptive pill can reduce absorption of B12. Vegans and vegetarians are more at risk of developing vitamin B12 deficiency because of their food choices.
	Deficiency symptoms include fatigue, pale complexion, breathlessness, mood swings, and poor memory and concentration.

Vitamin	**C (ascorbic acid)**
Function	Crucial for the growth and repair of cells, particularly collagen in connective tissue. It increases the body's natural resistance to infection.
Food sources	Fresh fruit (particularly citrus), berries, dried fruit, vegetables (dark green leafy vegetables, tomatoes and peppers, broccoli). However, a significant amount of vitamin C is lost in cooking.
Daily requirements	Children need 30mg / day, and adults 40mg / day.

Dangers of high doses	Excess is excreted in the urine, though high doses could result in diarrhoea and development of kidney stones. Avoid taking at levels above 1000mg / day.
Those at risk of deficiency	Poor healing, low resistance to infection.

Vitamin	**D**
Function	Supports the absorption of calcium from the intestine, and controls calcium metabolism and formation.
Food sources	Sunlight (UV), oily fish (herrings, sardines, mackerel, trout), eggs, margarines and some fortified breakfast cereals.
Daily requirements	People aged 4–64 years do not require a dietary source as long as their skin is exposed to sunlight.
Dangers of high doses	Toxicity is rare, but high intakes could lead to high blood pressure, irregular heartbeat and nausea.
Those at risk of deficiency	Deficiency symptoms include bone disorders, chronic muscle aches and pains.

Vitamin	**E**
Function	Protects body tissues against damage from free radicals, helps to form red blood cells, and supports normal growth and development.
Food sources	Pure vegetable oils, sunflower seeds, avocado, wholemeal bread and cereals. Meat, fish and eggs provide moderate amounts.
Daily requirements	4mg / day for men and 3mg / day for women.
Dangers of high doses	Toxicity is extremely rare.
Those at risk of deficiency	Low intakes may be associated with increased risk of coronary heart disease and degenerative conditions.

Mineral	Calcium
Function	Very important for strong and versatile bones and teeth.
	Also involved in muscle contraction and relaxation, blood clotting, and the transmission of nerve impulses.
Food sources	Low-fat dairy products, soft bones of small fish, fortified bread and white flour, green leafy vegetables, pulses, figs.
	NOTE: Some vegetables (e.g. spinach) contain oxalic acid, which reduces the absorption of calcium. Phytic acid in wholegrain cereals, nuts and pulses can also interfere with calcium absorption. Phosphoric acid in fizzy drinks significantly affects calcium absorption.
Daily requirements	Children (11–18 years) need 1000mg / day for boys, and 800mg / day for girls. Adults need 700mg / day.
Dangers of high doses	Very high intakes may interfere with the absorption of iron, and may also affect kidney function.
Those at risk of deficiency	Deficiency symptoms include cramps, fractures, muscles aches and uncontrolled twitching of leg muscles.

Mineral	Sodium
Function	Aids the balance of fluid in body tissues, and is involved in muscle contraction.
Food sources	Salt, meat, ready-made sauces, processed meats, savoury products (crisps, salted nuts), soups, bread.
Daily requirements	Intake usually far exceeds requirements, which are 69–460mg / day. Recommended maximum amount is 2.4g / day (equivalent to 6g of salt).

| **Dangers of high doses** | High salt intake may increase blood pressure and promote fluid retention. Excess salt could cause cramp (which can also be caused by dehydration and shortage of potassium). |
| **Those at risk of deficiency** | Excessive sweating (due to intense exercise and/or hot humid conditions) can cause substantial loss of sodium. |

Mineral	**Potassium**
Function	Works alongside sodium to control the balance of fluid in body tissues and support the contraction of muscle.
Food sources	Present in many foods, but very good sources include vegetables, fruit, fruit juices, wholegrain cereals, yeast extracts, milk, fish, eggs and dairy products.
Daily requirements	Adults require 3500mg / day.
Dangers of high doses	Excessive intake of potassium is excreted in the urine, and therefore toxicity is rare.
Those at risk of deficiency	Deficiency unlikely to occur through inadequate diet.

Mineral	**Iron**
Function	Involved in the synthesis of red blood cells (giving it a characteristic red colour) and aids the transport of oxygen around the body.
Food sources	Iron from animal sources is the best absorbed (red meat, liver, offal), and shellfish is another source.
	Wholegrain cereals, peas, beans and dried figs are also good sources of iron, but are poorly absorbed because phytates, also present in these foods, combine with iron and thus reduce its absorption.
	Iron is far better absorbed in the presence of vitamin C (found in fresh orange juice, fresh fruits, salads and vegetables).

Daily requirements	Males: 11–18 years require 11.3mg / day; 19 years and older require 8.7mg / day.
	Females: 11–50 years require 14.8mg / day; 50 years and older require 8.7mg / day.
Dangers of high doses	High doses may lead to stomach discomfort and constipation, and reduce the absorption of zinc. Avoid taking above 17mg / day.
Those at risk of deficiency	Symptoms of iron-deficiency anaemia include fatigue, pale complexion, headaches, hair loss and shortness of breath.
	Large quantities of strong tea (owing to its tannin content) can reduce iron absorption and thus increase the risk of deficiency.

Mineral	**Zinc**
Function	Widely involved in the metabolism of proteins, fats and carbohydrates.
	Crucial for wound healing and for protecting the body against infection.
Food sources	Good sources include meat, eggs, milk and dairy products. Wholegrain cereals, nuts and some vegetables also contain modest amounts of zinc, but the presence of oxalic acid and phytates reduces the availability of zinc in these particular foods.
Daily requirements	Over the age of 15 years, males require 9.5mg / day and females 7mg / day.
Dangers of high doses	High doses can lead to nausea and vomiting, and can interfere with the absorption of iron and other minerals.
Those at risk of deficiency	Deficiency symptoms include slow wound healing, acne, brittle nails and a lowered immune system. Zinc deficiency is common in dancers and in people who avoid meat and animal products.

Mineral	Magnesium
Function	Vital for the formation of new cells and for the contraction of muscles, and forms part of the mineral structure in bone.
Food sources	Available in virtually all foods, but good food sources include green vegetables, wholegrain cereals, muesli, vegetables, fruit, potatoes, milk and meat.
Daily requirements	300mg / day for men, 270mg / day for women.
Dangers of high doses	High doses may cause diarrhoea.
Those at risk of deficiency	Deficiency is unlikely. Symptoms include muscle weakness and cramps.

Mineral	Phosphorus
Function	Involved in the formation of healthy bones and teeth, and essential for the production of energy.
Food sources	Richest sources include meat, fish, milk and dairy products and green vegetables.
Daily requirements	Adults need around 550mg / day.
Dangers of high doses	High intakes over a short period of time can lead to stomach pains and diarrhoea, and over a longer time to lower blood calcium levels.
Those at risk of deficiency	Excessive quantities of alcohol can lower the absorption of phosphorus.

Essential and Non-essential Amino Acids

Essential

Histidine and Arginine are considered Essential for infants (not adults).

Isoleucine
Leucine
Valine
Lysine
Methionine
Phenylalanine
Threoline
Tryptophan
Histidine
Arginine

Semi-essential

Semi-essential amino acids are sometimes made internally if the conditions are right.

Cysteine
Tyrosine

Non-essential

Glycine
Proline
Glutamic Acid
Asparigine
Serine
Alanine
Aspartic Acid
Glutamine

Dance students at Laban Contemporary Dance in London undergo a screening
programme that evaluates the effectiveness of their training. Students experience
physiological, biomechanical and psychological assessments that determine their
readiness for the professional world of dance. The screening programme not only
incorporates conditioning programmes and advice to promote well-being and aid
the identification and prevention of injury, it also places great emphasis on
empowering dancers by encouraging them to embrace their own futures.
Photograph © Kyle Stevenson. Laban Contemporary Dance: London.

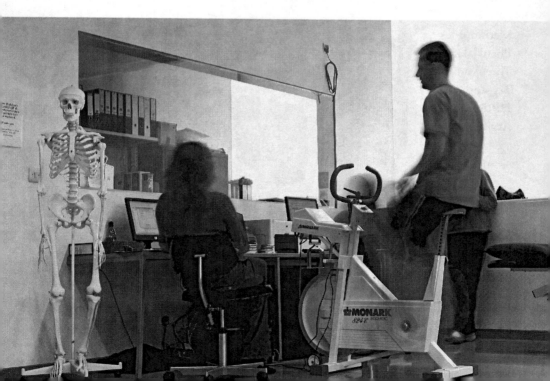

Appendix 8
Calculations

The following examples demonstrate how to calculate the right quantities of carbohydrate, protein and fat that comprise the balanced diet.

FAT = 25–30%
CARBOHYDRATE = 50–60%
PROTEIN = 15–20%

How much fat is needed in a 2000kcal diet?

To calculate 25% of a 2000 kcal diet:

$$\frac{2000kcal}{100\%} \text{ x25\% = 500kcal from fat}$$

To convert fat calories into grams (1 gram of fat = 9 kcal):

$$\frac{500kcal}{9} = 56g \text{ of fat}$$

To calculate 30% of a 2000 kcal diet:

$$\frac{2000kcal}{100\%} \text{ x30\% = 600kcal from fat}$$

To convert fat calories into grams (1 gram of fat = 9 kcal):

$$\frac{600\text{kcal}}{9} = 67\text{g of fat}$$

Therefore a dancer following a 2000 kcal diet should maintain a daily intake of 56–67g of fat.

How much carbohydrate is needed in a 2000kcal diet?

To calculate 50% of a 2000 kcal diet:

$$\frac{2000\text{kcal}}{100\%} \times 50\% = 1000\text{kcal from carbohydrate}$$

To convert carbohydrate calories into grams (1 gram of carbohydrate = 4 kcal):

$$\frac{1000\text{kcal}}{4} = 250\text{g of carbohydrate}$$

To calculate 60% of a 2000kcal diet:

$$\frac{2000\text{kcal}}{100\%} \times 60\% = 1200\text{kcal from carbohydrate}$$

To convert carbohydrate calories into grams (1 gram of carbohydrate = 4 kcal):

$$\frac{1200\text{kcal}}{4} = 300\text{g of carbohydrate}$$

Therefore a dancer following a 2000 kcal diet should maintain a daily intake of 250–300g of carbohydrate.

How much protein is needed in a 2000kcal diet?

To calculate 15% of a 2000 kcal diet:

$$\frac{2000\text{kcal}}{100\%} \times 15\% = 300\text{kcal from protein}$$

To convert protein calories into grams (1 gram of protein = 4 kcal):

$$\frac{300\text{kcal}}{4} = 75\text{g of protein}$$

To calculate 20% of a 2000kcal diet:

$$\frac{2000\text{kcal}}{100\%} \times 20\% = 400\text{kcal from protein}$$

To convert protein calories into grams (1 gram of protein = 4 kcal):

$$\frac{400\text{kcal}}{4} = 100\text{g of protein}$$

Therefore a dancer following a 2000 kcal diet should maintain a daily intake of 75–100g of protein.

Appendix 9
Weights and Measures

Height / Length

1 foot = 12 inches
1 foot = 0.305 m
1 inch = 0.0254 m
1 m = 39.37 inches

Weight / Mass

1 ounce (oz) = 28.35 grams (g)
1 pound (lb) = 16 ounces
1 pound = 0.45 kg
1 kg = 2.2 lb
1 stone (st) = 14 lb
1 stone = 6.35 kg

Appendix 10
References

Department of Health, *Dietary Reference Values for Food Energy and Nutrients for the United Kingdom*, Report of the Panel on Dietary Reference Values of the Committee on Medical Aspects of Food Policy (COMA) – Report on Health and Social Subjects 41, London, HMSO, 1991.

Food Standards Agency and Department of Health, *National Diet and Nutrition Survey of Adults Aged 19–64*, vol.5, London, HMSO, 2004.

Appendix 11
Further Reading

Ainsworth, B.E., Haskell, W.L., Whitt, M.C., Irwin, M.L., Swartz, A.M., Strath, S.J., O'Brien, W.L., Bassett, D.R.,Jr, Schmitz, K.H., Emplaincourt, P.O., Jacobs, D.R.,Jr, & Leon.A.S., 'Compendium of physical activities: an update of activity codes and MET intensities', *Medicine and Science in Sports and Exercise*, 32(9 Supplement), September 2000, pp. S498–S516.

Andreu, H., *Dance, Movement and Nutrition: Fitness Minutes for a Healthier Life*, Bloomington (Indiana), AuthorHouse, 2006.

Applegate, L., *Eat Smart, Play Hard*, Emmaus (Penn.), Rodale, 2001.

Bean, A., *The Complete Guide to Strength Training*, 3edn, London, A. & C. Black, 2005.

Bean, A., *Food for Fitness*, 2edn, London, A. & C. Black, 2002.

Bean, A., *The Complete Guide to Sports Nutrition*, 5edn, London, A. & C. Black, 2006).

Benardot, D., *Advanced Sports Nutrition*, Leeds, Human Kinetics, 2006.

Branner, T., *The Care and Feeding of a Dancer: What You Need to Know On and Off the Stage*, Waxhaw (N. Carolina), Blue Water Press, 2007.

Brinson, P. & Dick, F., *Fit to Dance? – The Report of the National Inquiry into Dancers' Health and Injury*, London, Dance UK, 1996.

Burke, L., & Deakin, V., *Clinical Sports Nutrition*, 3edn, London, McGraw-Hill, 2006.

Burke, L., *Practical Sports Nutrition*, Leeds, Human Kinetics, 2007.

Castelo-Branco, C., Reina, F., Montivero, A.D., Colodrón, M. & Vanrell, J.A., 'Influence of high-intensity training and of dietetic and anthropometric factors on menstrual cycle disorders in ballet dancers', *Gynecol Endocrinol*, Vol 22 No. 1, Jan. 2006, pp.31–5.

Chmelar, R.D. & Fitt, S.S., *Diet for Dancers: A Complete Guide to Nutrition and Weight Control*, Pennington (New Jersey), Princeton Book Company, 1995.

Clark, N., *Nancy Clark's Sports Nutrition Guidebook*, 4edn revised, Leeds, Human Kinetics Europe, 2008.

Franklin, E.N., *Conditioning for Dance*, Leeds, Human Kinetics, 2004.

Garrow, J.S., James, W.P.T. & Ralph, A., *Human Nutrition and Dietetics*, 10edn, Edinburgh, Churchill Livingstone, 2000.

Heyward, V.H. & Stolarczyk, L.M., *Applied Body Composition Assessment*, Leeds, Human Kinetics, 1996.

Howse, J., *Dance Technique and Injury Prevention*, 3edn, London, A. & C. Black, 2000.

Kreider, R.B., Fry, A.C. & O'Toole, M.L., *Overtraining in Sport*, Champaign (Illinois), Human Kinetics, 1998.

Laws, H., *Fit to Dance 2: The Report of the Second National Inquiry into Dancers' Health and Injury in the UK*, Dance UK, London, 2005.

Matthews, B.L., Bennell, K.L., McKay, H.A., Khan, K.M., Baxter-Jones, A.D., Mirwald, R.L. & Wark, J.D., 'Dancing for bone health: a 3-year longitudinal study of bone mineral accrual across puberty in female non-elite dancers and controls', *Osteoporosis Int*, Vol 17 No. 7, 2006, pp. 1043–54.

McArdle, W.D., Katch, F.I. & Katch, V.L., *Sports and Exercise Nutrition*, 3edn, Philadelphia (Penn.), Lippincott Williams and Wilkins, 2008).

McCance, R.A., Widdowson, E.M. & Holland, B., *McCance & Widdowson's Composition of Foods*, Royal Society of Chemistry, London, 1991.

Meltzer, S. & Fuller, C., *The Complete Book of Sports Nutrition: A Practical Guide to Eating for Sport*, London, New Holland, 2005.

Miller, C., 'Dance Medicine: Current Concepts', *Phys Med Rehabil Clin N Am*, Vol 17 No. 4, Nov. 2006, pp. 803–11.

Motta-Valencia, K., 'Dance-related Injury', *Phys Med Rehabil Clin N Am*, Vol 17 No. 3, Aug. 2006, pp. 697–723.

Noh, Y.E., Morris, T. & Andersen, M.B., 'Psychological Intervention Programs for Reduction of Injury in Ballet Dancers', *Res Sports Med*, Vol 15 No. 1, Jan.–Mar. 2007, pp.13–32.

Oreb, G., Ruzi, L., Matkovi, B., Misigoj-Durakovi, M., Vlasi, J. & Ciliga, D., 'Physical fitness, menstrual cycle disorders and smoking habit in Croatian National Ballet and National Folk Dance Ensembles', *Coll Antropol*, Vol 30 No. 2, June 2006, pp. 279–83.

Ravaldi, C., Vannacci, A., Bolognesi, E., Mancini, S., Faravelli, C. & Ricca, V., 'Gender role, eating disorder symptoms, and body image concern in ballet dancers', *J Psychosom Res*, Vol 61 No. 4, Oct. 2006, pp. 529–35.

Ringham, R., Klump, K., Kaye, W., Stone, D., Libman, S., Stowe, S. & Marcus, M., 'Eating disorder symptomatology among ballet dancers', *Int J Eat Disord*, Vol 39 No. 6, Sep. 2006, pp. 503–8.

Schoene, L.M., 'Biomechanical evaluation of dancers and assessment of their risk of injury', *J Am Podiatr Med Assoc*, Vol 97 No. 1, Jan.-Feb. 2007, pp. 75–80.

Stanfield, P.S., *Nutrition and Diet Therapy: Self-Instructional Modules*, 4edn, Boston, Jones and Bartlett, 2003.

To, W.W., Wong, M.W. & Lam, I.Y., 'Bone mineral density differences between adolescent dancers and non-exercising adolescent females', *J Pediatr Adolesc Gynecol*, Vol 18 No. 5, Oct. 2005, pp. 337–42.

To, W.W. & Wong, M.W., 'Comparison of quality of life scores among non-exercising adolescent females and adolescent dancers with oligomenorrhea and amenorrhea', *J Pediatr Adolesc Gynecol*, Vol 20 NO. 2, Apr. 2007, pp. 83–8.

Turner, B.S. & Wainwright, S.P., 'Corps de ballet: the case of the injured ballet dancer', *Social Health Illn*, Vol 25 No. 4, May 2003, pp. 269–88.

Urdapilleta, I., Cheneau, C., Masse, L. & Blanchet, A., 'Comparative study of body image among dancers and anorexic girls', *Eat Weight Disord*, Vol 12 No. 3, Sep. 2007, pp. 140–6.

Wainwright, S.P., Williams, C. & Turner, B.S., 'Fractured identities: injury and the balletic body', *Health (London)*, Vol 9 No. 1, Jan. 2005, pp. 49–66.

Webster-Gandy, J., Madden, A. & Holdsworth, M., *Oxford Handbook of Nutrition and Dietetics*, Oxford, Oxford University Press, 2006.

Useful Websites and Addresses

Arts Council of England
14 Great Peter Street
London SW1P 3NQ
www.artscouncil.org.uk

British Actors' Equity Association
Guild House
Upper St Martin's Lane
London WC2 9EG
www.equity.org.uk

British Association for Performing Arts Medicine (BAPAM)
4th Floor, Totara Park House
34–36 Gray's Inn Road
London WC1X 8HR
www.bapam.org.uk

British Association of Sport and Exercise Sciences (BASES)
Leeds Metropolitan University
Carnegie Faculty of Sport and Education
Fairfax Hall Headingley Campus
Beckett Park
Leeds LS6 3QS
www.bases.org.uk

British Dietetic Association
5th Floor, Charles House
148–9 Great Charles Street
Queensway
Birmingham B3 3HT
www.bda.uk.com

British Nutrition Foundation
High Holborn House
52–54 High Holborn
London WC1V 6RQ
www.nutrition.org.uk

Council for Dance Education and Training (CDET)
Riverside Studios
Hammersmith
London W6 9RL
www.cdet.org.uk

Dance Books Ltd
The Old Bakery
4 Lenten Street
Alton
Hampshire
GU34 1HG
www.dancebooks.co.uk

Dance UK
2nd Floor, Finsbury Town Hall
Roseberry Avenue
London EC1R 4QT
www.danceuk.org

Eating Disorders Association
1st Floor, Wensum House
103 Prince of Wales Road
Norwich NR1 1DW
www.edauk.com

Food Standards Agency
Room 621, Hannibal House
PO Box 30080
London SE1 6YA
www.foodstandards.gov.uk

National Osteoporosis Society
Camerton
Bath BA2 OPJ
www.nos.org.uk

National Resource Centre for Dance (NRCD)
University of Surrey
Guildford GU2 7XH
www.surrey.ac.uk/NRCD

National Sports Medicine Institute of the UK
32 Devonshire Street
London W1G 6PX
www.nsmi.org.uk

Nutrition Society
10 Cambridge Court
210 Shepherds Bush Road
London W6 7NJ
www.nutsoc.org

Vegetarian Society
Parkdale
Dunham Road
Altrincham WA14 4QG
www.vegsoc.org

Appendix 13
Journals and Magazines

All addresses are in the UK unless otherwise specified, and all phone and fax numbers are for calls originating in the UK.

Ballettanz
Editor: Franz Anton Cramer (English edition)
ReinhardtstraBe 29
D-10117 Berlin
Germany
Tel: 00 49 30 254 49520
Fax: 00 49 30 254 49524
www.ballet-tanz.de

Dance Europe
Editor: Emma Manning
P.O. Box 12661
London E5 9TZ
Tel: 0208 985 7767
Fax: 0208 525 0462
www.danceeurope.net

Dance Expression Magazine
Editor: Jean Rush
38 Ambleside Drive
Spalding PE11 1JU
Tel / Fax: 01775 712856
www.danceexpression.co.uk

Dance Gazette
Editor: David Jays
Royal Academy of Dance
36 Battersea Square
London SW11 3RA
Tel: 0207 326 8000
Fax: 0207 924 3129
www.rad.org.uk

Dance Magazine
Editor: Richard Phillip
111 Myrtle Street
Suite 203
Oakland
CA 94607
USA
Tel: 001 510 839 6060
Fax: 001 510 839 6066
www.dancemagazine.com

Dance Spirit
Editor: Laura Teusink
110 William Street
23rd Floor
New York
NY 10038
USA
Tel: 001 646 459 4800
Fax: 001 646 459 4900
www.dancespirit.com

Dance Teacher
Managing Editor: Jeni Tu
110 William Street
23rd Floor
New York
NY 10038
USA
Tel: 001 646 459 4800
Fax: 001 646 459 4900
www.dance-teacher.com

Dance Theatre Journal
Editor: Martin Hargreaves
LABAN
Creekside
London SE8 3DZ
Tel: 020 8691 8600
Fax: 020 8691 8400
www.laban.org/home/publications/_dance_theatre_journal.phtml

Dance Today
Editor: Katie Gregory
Clerkenwell House
45–47 Clerkenwell Green
London EC1R 0EB
Tel: 020 7250 3006
Fax: 020 7253 6679
www.dance-today.co.uk

Dance UK News
Editors: Catherine Willmore, Jeanette Siddall, Helen Laws
Battersea Arts Centre
Lavender Hill
London SW11 5TN
Tel: 0207 228 4990
Fax: 0207 223 0074
www.danceuk.org

Dancing Times
Editor: Jonathan Gray
Clerkenwell House
45–47 Clerkenwell Green
London EC1R 0EB
Tel: 0207 250 3006
Fax: 0207 253 6679
www.dancing-times.co.uk

Filmwaves
Editor: Marco Zee-Jotti
PO Box 420
Edgware HA8 420
www.filmwaves.co.uk

Journal of Dance Medicine and Science
Editors-in-chief: Karen S. Clippinger, M.S.P.E., Scott E. Brown, M.D.
J. Michael Ryan Publishing Inc.
24 Crescent Drive North
Andover
NJ 07821-4000
USA
Tel: 001 973 786 7777
Fax: 001 973 786 7776
www.iadms.org/displaycommon.cfm?an=1&subarticlenbr=47

Juice Magazine
The Place Artist Development
17 Duke's Road
London WC1H 9PY
Tel: 020 7387 1828
fax: 020 7388 5407
www.theplace.org.uk

Pointe
Editor: Virginia Johnson
110 William Street
23rd Floor
New York
NY 10038
USA
Tel: 001 646 459 4800
Fax: 001 646 459 4900
www.pointemagazine.com

Pulse Magazine
Editor: Chitra Sundaram
Asian Dance & Music Ltd
1 Lurke Street
Bedford MK40 3TN
Tel: 01234 316 028
www.kadam.org.uk/pulse.php

The Stage
Editor: Brian Atwood
Stage House
47 Bermondsey Street
London SE1 3XT
Tel: 0207 403 1818
Fax: 0207 357 9287
www.thestage.co.uk

Theatregoer Magazine
Editor: Ruth Leon
11 Plough Yard
London EC2A 3LP
Tel: 01752 312 140
Fax: 01752 313 162
www.reallyuseful.com/theatregoer

*Total Theatre Magazine (*including *Circus News)*
Editor: John Daniel
Total Theatre Network
The Power Station
Coronet Street
London N1 6HD
Tel: 0207 729 7944
Fax: 0207 729 7945
www.circusarts.org.uk

Index

9 781852 731359